My Child Has Scoliosis

Dr. Juan Jesus Villa

My Child Has Scoliosis:

A Mother's Guide to Understanding their Child's Journey

Dr. Juan Jesus Villa

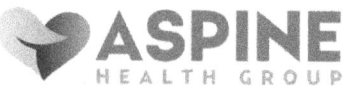

ASPINE Health Group Inc. Publishing

My Child Has Scoliosis

My Child Has Scoliosis: A Mother's Guide to Understanding Their Journey

For permission requests, contact:
ASPINE Health Group Inc.
A nonprofit organization dedicated to posture and scoliosis education
Email: aspinehealth@gmail.com

ISBN: 979-8-218-83133-2
Issued in the United States of America

First Edition – 2026

Cover design by Dr. Juan Jesus Villa
Published by **ASPINE Health Group Inc.**

Disclaimer:
This book is intended for informational and educational purposes only. It is not a substitute for professional medical advice, diagnosis, or treatment. Always seek the advice of your physician or other qualified health provider regarding any medical condition or treatment.

Dr. Juan Jesus Villa

Table of Contents

ABOUT THE AUTHOR 5
ACKNOWLEDGMENTS 7
THE REASON THIS BOOK WAS WRITTEN 9

SECTION 1: DOES YOUR CHILD HAVE SCOLIOSIS?.... 12

1. UNDERSTANDING SCOLIOSIS 12
2. DIFFERENT TYPES OF SCOLIOSIS.......................................15
3. DETECTING SCOLIOSIS...20
4. WHERE WILL THEIR SCOLIOSIS JOURNEY TAKE THEM NEXT? 24

SECTION 2: THE PAIN OF SCOLIOSIS 27

5. PHYSICAL PAIN FROM SCOLIOSIS.......................................27
6. THE EMOTIONAL PAIN OF SCOLIOSIS 30
7. MANAGING THEIR SCOLIOSIS 32
8. THE REAL CONSEQUENCES OF LIFE WITH SCOLIOSIS 35
9. NAVIGATING LIFE WITH SCOLIOSIS 37
10. WHAT TO EXPECT IF SCOLIOSIS IS NOT ADDRESSED? 39
11. IT'S NEVER GOING TO GET BETTER ON ITS OWN 41

SECTION 3: CAN YOU DO SOMETHING ABOUT THEIR SCOLIOSIS? 43

12. WHAT DOES SUCCESSFUL TREATMENT LOOKS LIKE? 43
13. GETTING ON THE SAME PAGE WITH PEOPLE WHO CAN HELP 45
14. ARE YOUR PROVIDERS SPECIALIZED IN SCOLIOSIS? 48
15. A PICTURE OF WHAT'S POSSIBLE 51

SECTION 4: SHOULD YOUR CHILD HAVE SCOLIOSIS SURGERY? 53

16. WHAT IS IT LIKE TO HAVE SPINAL FUSION SURGERY FOR SCOLIOSIS? 53

17. SURGERY CREATES A NEW NORMAL: WHAT WILL THAT MEAN FOR THEM? 56

18. SURGERY ISN'T THE END OF SCOLIOSIS 60

SECTION 5: EFFECTIVE SCOLIOSIS TREATMENT 67

20. SCOLIOSIS-SPECIFIC CHIROPRACTIC 67

21. UNDERSTANDING SPINAL TRACTION IN SCOLIOSIS MANAGEMENT 73

    Decompression Traction... 73

    Structural Traction.. 74

22. SCOLIOSIS-BRACING 78

23. WHAT RESULTS TO EXPECT FROM TREATMENT? 86

24: YOU HAVE CONTROL 90

QUESTIONS YOU CAN ASK YOUR CHILD'S DOCTOR ABOUT THEIR SCOLIOSIS DIAGNOSIS 94

HELPFUL RESOURCES 99

POSTURE CHECKLIST 100

RECOMMENDED EXERCISES DEPENDING ON THEIR UNIQUE CURVE...102

REFERENCE SECTION 103

About the Author

Dr. Juan Jesus Villa's journey began in the small community of Heber in the Imperial Valley, California, where he first witnessed the profound challenges faced by individuals battling chronic health issues. Inspired by these early experiences and driven by an unwavering desire to make a meaningful difference, he pursued advanced studies in rehabilitation and chiropractic care.

This passion led him to co-found **ASPINE Health Group**, a nonprofit organization dedicated to helping individuals with spinal ailments, and to serve as the Chief Medical Officer at Xuyang Doctor's Group in China, all while establishing himself as a respected university lecturer in spinal biomechanics, posture correction, and scoliosis management.

Throughout his distinguished career, Dr. Juan has devoted himself to understanding and mitigating the effects of scoliosis. His extensive hands-on experience managing complex cases, combined with significant contributions to scientific literature, has shaped his compassionate, evidence-based approach to care.

At the core of Dr. Juan's philosophy is his signature concept: **Posture-Full®**.

More than a brand, *Posture-Full®* is a mindset, a way of living with awareness, alignment, and intention. It reflects Dr. Juan's belief that posture is more than how we stand or sit; it is a window into how we feel, function, and grow.

Being **Posture-Less** means living unaware, unsupported, and unprepared.
Being **Posture-Full®** means living empowered understanding your body, making better decisions, and actively investing in your long-term health.

Today, Dr. Juan's work stands as a beacon of hope and guidance for families navigating the intricacies of scoliosis, with a steadfast emphasis on early intervention, lifelong wellness, and becoming **Posture-Full®** in every stage of life.

Dr. Juan

POSTURE-FULL® CHIRO

Acknowledgments

I extend my deepest gratitude to all my patients and their devoted mothers who have placed their trust in me throughout their scoliosis journeys. Allowing me to walk alongside your family during such a vulnerable and uncertain time is an honor I do not take lightly. Each conversation, each appointment, and each decision you have entrusted to me has pushed me to grow, to learn, and to continually raise the standard of care I strive to provide.

Your courage, resilience, and unwavering commitment in the face of fear and unanswered questions have been nothing short of extraordinary. I have witnessed the emotional weight you carry as parents and the strength you summon day after day to advocate for your children. Watching you persevere through difficult choices, celebrate small victories, and remain present even in moments of exhaustion has deeply shaped not only my clinical approach, but also my understanding of what true healing truly means.

This book is not only a reflection of my dedication to scoliosis care, but a tribute to every family who shows up daily with hope, discipline, and love. Your willingness to seek answers, act, and believe in the possibility of improvement even when the future feels uncertain is the reason this work exists.

To Gina, my wife, thank you for choosing to walk this journey with me. Your support has never been passive or automatic. It has been a deliberate and self-giving decision to believe in the mission we share. In choosing to stand beside me, you chose the long hours, the uncertainty, and the responsibility that comes with serving others. What some might call sacrifice, I recognize as an act of intentional love. One that has strengthened both my work and my purpose. You are not only my partner in life, but a constant reminder of why this work matters.

Above all, I give thanks to God, whose guidance has shaped every step of this journey. In moments of doubt, He provided clarity. In moments of fatigue, He renewed my strength. This work, this book, and the lives it hopes to impact are all possible because of His inspiration, grace, and calling.

Dr. Juan Jesus Villa

The reason this book was written

As a parent, hearing the diagnosis of scoliosis for your child is like being thrust into a stormy sea with no lifeboat in sight. It's a moment that freezes time, where the world seems to come crashing down around you. You're suddenly faced with a reality you never imagined, one filled with uncertainty and fear. Every parent's worst nightmare is seeing their child suffer, and scoliosis embodies that fear in its very essence.

The image of your child's spine twisting and bending, pressing against vital organs, sends shivers down your spine. It's a relentless weight that bears down on your shoulders, threatening to suffocate you with its magnitude.

In those initial moments, you feel lost, overwhelmed by the sheer magnitude of what lies ahead. Questions swarm your mind like relentless bees, each one buzzing louder than the last. What does this mean for their future? Will they be in pain? How will this impact their quality of life? But what if I told you it doesn't have to be a death sentence?

There is hope. It's the realization that you're not alone in this journey. You find strength in the love you have for your child, a force more powerful than any diagnosis. With every tear shed and every sleepless night endured, you resolve to be their unwavering support, their guiding light through the darkness.

9

What if there was a way to not just endure, but to actively combat this condition?

Scoliosis is simply a curvature of the spine measuring more than 10° from the front. As our children grow, their spines can develop these sideways bends. In most cases, the curvature stays under 20°. It's a natural phenomenon; a sideways bend that can occur as children grow. Often, these curves remain mild, staying under 20°, and conventional wisdom advises waiting until they worsen significantly before considering surgery. But what if I told you there are other options? What if I told you there's a way to fight back, and take control?

You don't have to watch helplessly as a 15° curve grows into a 40° nightmare. You can act now. Hope is a powerful force. It's the fuel that drives us forward, even in our darkest moments. And I know, in this moment, you're scared. You're overwhelmed with questions and doubts. Every internet search only adds to the confusion. In the face of scoliosis, you don't have to be a helpless bystander, watching as a 15° curve spirals into a 40° nightmare. The power to act lies within your grasp, and hope serves as your guiding light, illuminating the path forward even in the darkest of moments.

That's the reason why I wrote this book. Through my years of dedicated practice in spinal correction, I've been privileged to witness miracles unfold before my eyes. I've seen children's spines undergo incredible

10

transformations, defying the odds stacked against them. But I've also borne witness to the devastation wrought by the rapid deterioration of untreated scoliosis. It's a relentless race against time, one where every moment counts, demanding swift and decisive action.

You are not alone in this journey. Together, armed with knowledge and fueled by determination, we can confront scoliosis head-on and rewrite its story. This book is more than just a collection of words; it's a beacon of hope, a roadmap to empowerment in the face of adversity. Within its pages, you'll find the tools and insights needed to navigate the complexities of scoliosis treatment with confidence and clarity.

Section 1: Does your child have Scoliosis?

1. Understanding Scoliosis

Scoliosis is when the spine bends sideways, forming a C-shape or S-shape instead of staying straight. Doctors use special pictures called X-rays to check the spine's bend, which is considered significant if it's more than 10 degrees. This bend can occur anywhere along the spine, from the neck to the lower back, and its severity can vary from person to person. Don't worry about radiation – nowadays, X-rays are advanced and expose you to about the same amount of radiation as you'd encounter during a long flight. So, while it's important to monitor the spine's curve, there's no need for concern about the X-ray process itself.

Scoliosis can affect anyone, from babies to adults. While we're not always sure why it happens, there are different reasons that might play a part. Sometimes, scoliosis is there from the start because of how the spine formed before birth. Other times, it might be because of certain conditions like cerebral palsy or muscular dystrophy, which can affect how our muscles work and lead to a curved spine.

Most of the time, though, we don't know exactly why scoliosis happens. This is called idiopathic scoliosis, and it usually shows up during the teenage years. It's more common in girls than boys, and while genetics

12

might have something to do with it, things like how we grow during puberty could also play a part. One of the reasons scoliosis is more commonly diagnosed in girls often at an earlier stage than boys is because girls grow and develop faster. If you take a 12-year-old girl and a 12-year-old boy, in most cases, the girl will be taller. This is because girls tend to hit their growth spurts earlier, with rapid skeletal growth occurring before boys begin their major growth phases. This accelerated growth plays a significant role in scoliosis development.

Growth plates, which are the soft areas at the ends of bones where growth occurs, close earlier in girls than in boys. For most girls, this closure happens between the ages of 14 and 16, whereas boys typically continue growing until their growth plates close around 16 to 18 years old. Since scoliosis progression is most aggressive during rapid growth phases, girls often experience spinal curve progression sooner than boys.

This is why early detection is so crucial. So, whether you're young or old, understanding that scoliosis can happen to anyone is important. While the exact reasons may not always be clear, early detection and proper treatment can significantly improve how scoliosis impacts our lives.

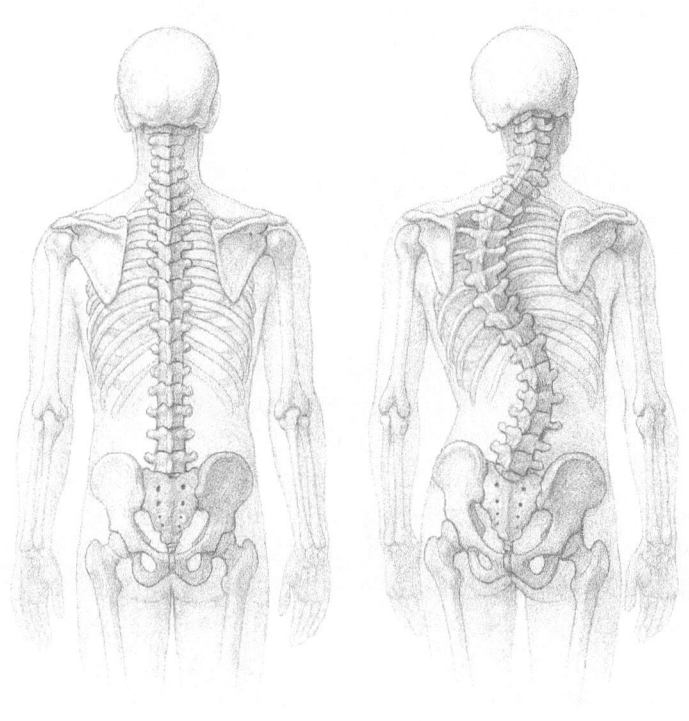

*Left side shows a normal spine. The right figure
demonstrates a scoliotic spine.*

2. Different Types of Scoliosis

a. Congenital Scoliosis: When your baby's spine doesn't develop properly before birth, it can lead to a condition called congenital scoliosis. Some spinal bones might be misshapen, resembling butterflies or wedges. More than just physical irregularities, these signs can sometimes point to broader developmental issues, requiring careful and comprehensive medical attention. Think of it as building a tower with blocks, if one block is out of place, it affects the whole structure.

Similarly, these abnormal formations in the spine can cause significant curvature and misalignment. Treatment varies greatly with the severity, ranging from regular monitoring to more active interventions like bracing or surgery. As parents, your close collaboration with pediatricians and orthopedic surgeons is crucial to tailor the treatment that best fits your child's needs.

b. Neuromuscular Scoliosis: Imagine the struggle of keeping a stack of books balanced on a shaky table. For children with conditions like cerebral palsy or muscular dystrophy, their muscles don't support their spine well, which can cause it to bend improperly. This type of scoliosis makes moving around not just difficult but often painful.

Managing this condition may involve exercises specifically designed to strengthen muscles and improve posture, or in more severe cases, surgery might be necessary to realign and stabilize the spine.

The treatment aims to maintain as much spinal functionality as possible, reducing discomfort and enhancing mobility.

c. Degenerative Scoliosis: Often seen in adults over the age of 40 or 50, degenerative scoliosis occurs as the spine naturally ages and undergoes changes, including the degeneration of discs and joints. This progression can be exacerbated by conditions like osteoarthritis. The gradual flattening of the lumbar curve, a critical factor in weight distribution and spinal alignment, can lead to the spine compensating in other areas, causing it to twist and curve.

Early intervention, focusing on maintaining proper posture and employing specialized exercises, can be incredibly beneficial in managing symptoms and slowing the condition's progression.

d. Idiopathic Scoliosis: The most prevalent form of scoliosis typically emerges during the teenage years, coinciding with periods of rapid growth. The term 'idiopathic' means the exact cause is unknown, which can be particularly frustrating for both you and your child. This condition can range from mild, where it's barely noticeable, to severe cases that might require bracing or surgery. Regular monitoring is essential, as early detection allows for interventions that can significantly improve the quality of life and reduce the need for more invasive treatments.

Imagine waking up one day and noticing that your child's back isn't as straight as it used to be. That's what happens with idiopathic scoliosis, the most common type of scoliosis, and it often shows up during the teenage years, between 10 and 18 years old. It's like a mysterious guest that arrives uninvited, leaving parents and children alike scratching their heads in confusion.

Doctors use the word "idiopathic" to describe this type of scoliosis because, well, they don't really know what causes it. It's like a puzzle with missing pieces, leaving experts puzzled about what triggers the spine to start curving. Some researchers think it might have something to do with our genes, like passing down a tendency to develop a curved spine from one generation to the next. Others wonder if it's linked to growth spurts during adolescence, when the body grows rapidly. Other factors can be link to lifestyle and poor posture.

Despite the mystery surrounding its origins, doctors have learned a lot about idiopathic scoliosis over the years. They've found that it's not just one condition but rather a group of curves that behave differently depending on when they start and how severe they are. There are curves that appear early, known as juvenile scoliosis, and curves that show up later, during the teenage years, called adolescent scoliosis. Some curves stay small and don't cause much trouble, while others grow larger and can lead to problems with posture, breathing, and even self-esteem.

But here's some good news: just because idiopathic scoliosis is a bit of a mystery doesn't mean it's impossible to manage.

In fact, doctors have a whole arsenal of tools and treatments to help keep those curves in check. For mild curves, they might recommend regular check-ups to monitor how things are going and maybe a bit of physical therapy to strengthen the muscles around the spine. For more severe curves, they might suggest wearing a brace to support the spine as it grows or even surgery to straighten things out.

e. Functional Scoliosis: Unlike the structural changes seen in other types of scoliosis, functional scoliosis arises from external factors, such as a discrepancy in leg length or muscle imbalances. This can tilt the pelvis and cause compensatory spinal curvature.

Thankfully, this type of scoliosis is often reversible, with treatments aimed at addressing the underlying cause, such as orthotics for leg length discrepancy, or short leg and physical therapy to strengthen and balance muscles.

The encouraging news for parents is that functional scoliosis is not a permanent condition and can often be effectively managed or even completely corrected. Treatment typically focuses on addressing the root cause. This might involve customized exercises designed to strengthen weak muscles and stretch tight ones, ensuring that the spine is supported evenly.

Physical therapy can also play a key role by teaching your child proper body mechanics and posture. In cases where leg length discrepancy is the culprit, specially fitted shoe inserts or orthotics can help balance the pelvis and realign the spine.

Navigating the complexities of scoliosis can be daunting, but understanding the nuances of each type helps you advocate for and support your child through their treatment journey. Whether dealing with a congenital issue present at birth or managing conditions that develop later, knowing what steps to take can provide reassurance and a path forward during challenging times.

So, while idiopathic scoliosis may be a mystery, it's a mystery that doctors and families can work together to solve. With early detection, regular check-ups, and a bit of teamwork, there's no curve too big to conquer.

3. Detecting Scoliosis

Before considering any treatment options for your child, confirming the presence of scoliosis is crucial. Detecting this condition can often begin with something as simple as observing your child's posture during daily activities. Signs such as asymmetries in how they stand, or walk can serve as early indicators.

For instance, you might notice one shoulder appearing higher than the other, an unbalanced stance, or an uneven gait where your child sways more to one side. Even the way their clothes fit one side of a shirt such as hanging lower or a jacket not sitting evenly can provide clues.

Further assessments are often carried out in school settings. The Adams Forward Bend Test, frequently conducted during school physicals, involves the child bending forward from the waist with feet together. The appearance of a rib hump on one side is a sign of scoliosis, indicating a rotation in the spine.

Additionally, a tool called a scolio-meter might be used to measure the angle of trunk rotation. A reading of 5 degrees or more is generally a prompt for a more definitive examination, such as an X-ray.

Diagnostic imaging, such as X-rays, provides concrete confirmation of scoliosis. The measurement of the Cobb angle is essential here, it quantifies the degree of spinal curvature, with an angle of 10 degrees or more confirming the diagnosis. Another important assessment from X-ray images is the Risser Sign, which evaluates skeletal maturity by examining the ossification status of the iliac crest. This helps in predicting the potential for further progression of the spinal curve, which is pivotal in guiding treatment decisions.

Concerns about radiation exposure from X-rays are common, especially for children. However, modern X-ray technology utilizes very low levels of radiation, and precautions such as shielding reproductive organs are routinely employed to ensure safety. The benefits of accurately diagnosing and managing scoliosis far outweigh the minimal risks associated with these X-rays.

Screening for scoliosis is particularly critical between the ages of 12 to 14, a period that coincides with significant growth spurts in children. Girls typically experience these spurts around 11 to 12 years old and boys a bit later, around 13 to 14 years old. During this time, the spine grows rapidly, which can significantly accentuate any existing scoliosis or reveal previously undetected cases.

Early detection allows for interventions such as bracing, which are most effective before the spine reaches full maturity. These early interventions can often prevent the condition from worsening, potentially avoiding the need for surgical solutions later.

Moreover, early adolescence is a delicate period both physically and emotionally. Managing scoliosis effectively during these formative years can prevent physical discomfort and the emotional distress associated with more visible signs and symptoms of the condition.

Adolescents are particularly conscious of their physical appearance and how they are perceived by their peers. Timely and effective treatment can thus boost their self-esteem and mitigate any potential social or psychological challenges.

Thus, regular screenings during this pivotal developmental stage are not merely precautionary, they are essential. It ensures that any signs of scoliosis are managed promptly and effectively, thereby safeguarding not only the physical health of children but also their overall well-being and quality of life.

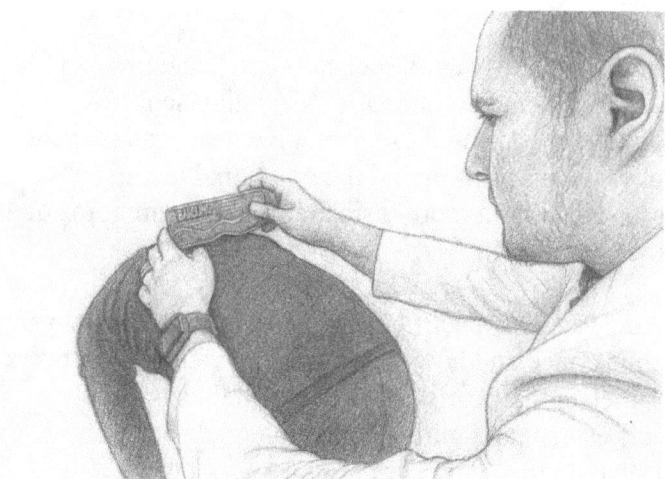

Illustration shows a doctor performing the routine Adams Test (scoliosis screening test).

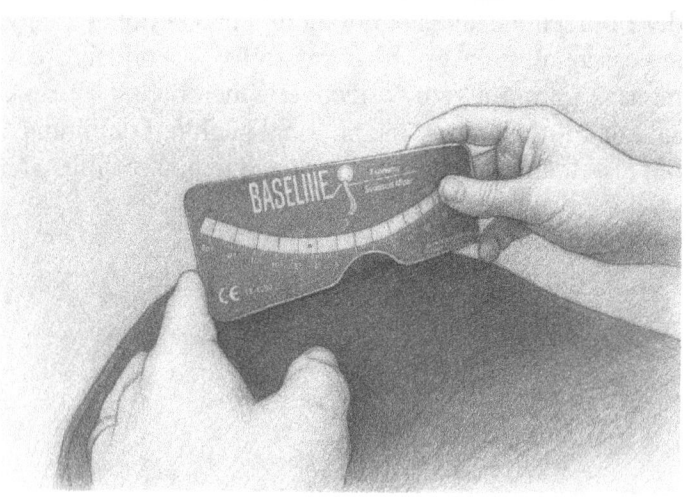

Illustration shows a scolio-meter to check the degrees of the back hump.

4. Where Will Their Scoliosis Journey Take Them Next?

Living with scoliosis is a journey filled with twists and turns, challenges, and triumphs. For those diagnosed with scoliosis, the path ahead may seem uncertain, yet with the right guidance and support, it's entirely possible to navigate this journey with confidence and resilience.

The journey often starts with that initial diagnosis, a moment that can feel daunting and overwhelming for individuals and their families. Suddenly, there are a myriad of questions: What will the progression of the curvature look like? Will it worsen over time? What treatment options are available? The uncertainty can stir up anxiety and fear as they step onto this unfamiliar path.

After receiving a diagnosis, the next step is to decide to seek professional help. This crucial decision, and the details of what it entails, will be covered more comprehensively in later chapters.
Understanding when and how to seek professional guidance is fundamental in managing the condition effectively.

As the journey unfolds, a variety of treatment options come into play, ranging from conservative methods like bracing and physical therapy to more invasive procedures such as surgery. Each decision requires careful consideration, balancing the risks and benefits of various treatment approaches to find the best fit for the individual's needs and preferences.

Throughout their journey, individuals with scoliosis might face physical and emotional ups and downs. Treatments and adjustments to living with scoliosis can bring about pain, discomfort, and mobility limitations. Simultaneously, they might deal with feelings of self-consciousness, isolation, and anxiety that impact their mental and emotional well-being.

Amidst these challenges, the journey is also marked by profound moments of resilience, strength, and personal growth. Individuals learn to adapt to their condition, discovering effective ways to manage symptoms and overcome obstacles with determination and perseverance. They tap into an inner strength they may not have known they had, developing a renewed appreciation for their bodies and capabilities.

Empowerment often becomes a key theme as they advance in their journey, with individuals becoming advocates for their own health and well-being. They learn to seek out and utilize resources, connect with supportive networks, and engage healthcare providers who understand their unique needs and can offer the necessary guidance and assistance.

Ultimately, the scoliosis journey isn't about reaching a destination but about the ongoing process of growth and self-discovery. It's a path filled with hope, resilience, and a steadfast belief that no matter the challenges ahead, they have the strength and courage to face them head-on and emerge stronger and more resilient than ever before.

Section 2: The pain of scoliosis

5. *Physical Pain from Scoliosis*

Living with scoliosis can be physically challenging, and the impact of the condition changes with age. The abnormal curvature of the spine places a constant strain on muscles and ligaments, leading to an uneven distribution of body weight. This imbalance is exacerbated by gravity, which pulls continuously on the misaligned spine, forcing certain muscle groups to exert extra effort to maintain stability. Over time, this overexertion can cause the muscles to become overworked and fatigued, weaving persistent discomfort and stiffness into daily life.

During childhood, the physical manifestations of scoliosis are typically mild, with most patients experiencing only minimal or intermittent discomfort that rarely disrupts their routine. The pain is often a subtle background noise, easily drowned out by the vibrant energy of youth. However, as individuals transition from childhood into adolescence and then adulthood, the cumulative effects of gravity on the curved spine become more pronounced.

The muscles that have been compensating for the spinal misalignment begin to wear out, leading to deeper, more persistent aches and a noticeable decrease in flexibility.

This gradual progression highlights the crucial role of early intervention and regular monitoring. While children may appear active and pain-free, ongoing assessment is essential to manage scoliosis proactively. Implementing early interventions, such as gentle stretching, postural exercises, and targeted physical therapy, can lay a solid foundation for healthier musculoskeletal development. Encouraging activities that strengthen the core and enhance flexibility is particularly beneficial, helping to support the spine more effectively.

Regular check-ups with a specialist are vital to ensure that any new or worsening symptoms are caught early, potentially delaying or lessening the severity of pain in adulthood. Although simple actions like bending to tie shoelaces or sitting for extended periods might eventually cause discomfort, these issues tend to emerge more prominently in later years, providing ample time to prepare and build resilience.

Understanding why scoliosis causes pain can also be enlightening. The spine's abnormal curvature disrupts the natural balance and alignment of the body, placing increased stress on the vertebrae and soft tissues. Over time, this stress can lead to inflammation, nerve compression, and changes in the joints and discs, all of which contribute to pain and functional limitations.

It's important to note that while scoliosis is more commonly diagnosed in children and adolescents, the physical pains associated with it are more likely to affect adults. This delayed onset of symptoms underscores the importance of continuous care throughout one's life. By staying informed about the potential progression of scoliosis and maintaining an active involvement in treatment strategies, individuals can manage their condition effectively and minimize the impact on their quality of life.

The good news is that regular chiropractic care can play a significant role in managing the pain associated with scoliosis. Chiropractic techniques, which focus on improving spinal alignment and function, can help alleviate the stress on the musculoskeletal system caused by scoliosis. Regular chiropractic adjustments, combined with a comprehensive treatment plan, can significantly reduce discomfort, improve mobility, and enhance overall well-being for those living with scoliosis.

6. The Emotional Pain of Scoliosis

The emotional toll of scoliosis can be just as challenging as the physical aspects of the condition. During adolescence, a period already filled with social and self-esteem challenges, the impact of a visible spinal deformity can be particularly magnified. While young children may not fully grasp or internalize these feelings, the most intense emotional distress often emerges during the teenage years and into adulthood.

For many teenagers, scoliosis becomes more than just a medical diagnosis; it transforms into a daily reminder of being different. The visible curvature of the spine can attract unwelcome attention or even hurtful comments, intensifying feelings of isolation and self-doubt. If not addressed early, this emotional burden may lead to chronic anxiety, deep-seated shame, and even depression.

It's important to understand that scoliosis is a journey, not a destination. Since scoliosis is a progressively changing condition, there isn't a cure but rather ways to manage, improve and monitor it. Emotional experiences will vary; sometimes, a new set of X-rays will show great improvement, while other times, they may not be so promising. These ups and downs are a natural part of managing scoliosis.

Frequent medical appointments, the necessity of wearing a brace, or even the prospect of surgical interventions contribute to a constant reminder of the condition. Each visit or treatment can reinforce a child's sense of vulnerability, impacting their self-image and self-worth. These experiences, compounded over time, can hinder the development of a healthy self-identity, making it crucial to address the emotional side of scoliosis.

Creating an environment where your child feels heard, understood, and supported is vital. Open conversations about the condition, along with professional counseling and support groups, can empower your child to express their feelings and learn coping strategies from peers facing similar challenges. By fostering self-acceptance and resilience from an early age, you can help mitigate the long-term emotional impact of scoliosis.

While the most intense emotional distress often manifests later in life, the seeds of self-doubt and insecurity are planted early. Proactive, compassionate support during childhood can ensure that when these feelings arise in adolescence and adulthood, your child is equipped with the strength and confidence to face them.

This understanding, that scoliosis is a continually evolving condition, underscores the importance of regular monitoring and adaptation of treatment strategies. It is a path filled with challenges, but with the right support and strategies, it is one that can be navigated successfully, allowing individuals to lead fulfilling lives despite the hurdles scoliosis may bring.

7. Managing Their Scoliosis

While there is no magic cure for scoliosis, a range of treatment options is available to help manage its symptoms and significantly improve the quality of life. The primary goal of these treatments isn't to simply eradicate discomfort overnight, but to alleviate pain and prevent the condition from worsening over time. For children, especially, conservative management often proves highly effective, as most of the intense pain associated with scoliosis tends to develop later in life.

Spinal rehabilitation plays a crucial role in managing scoliosis. It's not just about easing current discomfort, but also about building a solid foundation for long-term spine health. Exercise regimens designed by professionals experienced in pediatric scoliosis focus on building core strength, enhancing flexibility, and teaching proper body mechanics. These exercises are pivotal as they help reduce muscle strain and improve posture, enabling your child to remain active and comfortable while also preparing their body for future challenges.

Chiropractic care can complement physical therapy, by providing gentle adjustments aimed at alleviating nerve pressure and enhancing spinal alignment. Though, these adjustments are typically part of a broader treatment strategy rather than a standalone solution, many families find that regular and targeted care significantly reduces discomfort. These chiropractic interventions do more than relieve pain; they also play a critical role in preventing the progression of the curvature.

When conservative measures are not sufficient, additional pain management options may be necessary. Under careful medical supervision, options such as pain medications or even minimally invasive injections can offer temporary relief during periods of heightened discomfort. It is important to note that these methods are generally reserved for cases where other treatments have not yielded adequate results and are more commonly employed in adult patients experiencing severe symptoms.

In some scenarios, particularly when the curvature is pronounced and persistent, pain defies a comprehensive treatment plan; surgical interventions might be considered. The prospect of surgery can be daunting and is usually regarded as a last resort. Surgical options are generally postponed until adulthood, when the condition has had more time to progress, and the risk of severe pain and complications increases. By initiating early, conservative treatments tailored to your child's specific needs, you are actively working to delay or even prevent the onset of more severe pain later in life.

Ultimately, managing scoliosis is a journey, a proactive layered approach that evolves over time. By incorporating physical rehabilitation, chiropractic care, and when necessary, medical interventions you can help ensure that your child enjoys a higher quality of life today while building resilience for tomorrow. This multifaceted approach not only addresses current symptoms but also lays the groundwork for long-term well-being, giving both you and your child the confidence to face the future with strength and optimism.

Remember, scoliosis is a condition that progresses, and while it may not have a cure, it can be effectively managed with the right strategies, ensuring that each step forward is a step towards a healthier, more vibrant life.

8. The Real Consequences of Life with Scoliosis

If scoliosis remains untreated or progresses unchecked, it can lead to severe health complications over time. A significant spinal curvature can compress internal organs, leading to a range of critical issues that affect the body's fundamental functions. Respiratory difficulties may arise as the lungs find less room to expand, while digestive problems can occur due to the compression of the gastrointestinal tract. Moreover, severe scoliosis can impact cardiovascular function by exerting pressure on the heart, potentially leading to reduced cardiac efficiency.

These complications are more likely to manifest in later life, making early detection and proactive management during childhood crucial. The risks associated with untreated scoliosis aren't just limited to physical health. The condition can also severely affect an individual's quality of life, leading to chronic pain and significant physical limitations. This can inhibit daily activities, reduce participation in social and recreational activities, and impact mental health due to increased stress and anxiety about one's health and appearance.

Understanding these severe outcomes highlights the critical importance of a consistent and proactive treatment plan. Regular monitoring with healthcare professionals is essential to track the progression of the curvature and implement timely interventions. Parents should be vigilant about the warning signs, such as a noticeable increase in the curvature, worsening back pain, or symptoms indicating respiratory or cardiovascular strain. Maintaining a comprehensive record of your child's medical history and treatment progress is crucial for informed decision-making.

Early intervention can significantly mitigate these risks, helping your child maintain not only their physical health but also their ability to engage fully in life's activities. This proactive approach provides a solid foundation for a healthier future, dramatically reducing the likelihood of severe complications that could seriously compromise overall quality of life.

Adopting this informed and attentive approach to scoliosis management ensures that despite the challenges posed by this condition, individuals can lead active, fulfilling lives, minimizing the impact of scoliosis on their overall health and well-being.

9. Navigating Life with Scoliosis

Living with scoliosis often involves adapting to a life where modifications are necessary to manage pain and maintain function. These adjustments, whether it's opting for ergonomic furniture, making conscious efforts to maintain proper posture, or incorporating regular exercise into a busy schedule, are not signs of weakness or defeat. Instead, they are empowering strategies that effectively manage the condition over the long term.

It is crucial to teach your child how to navigate these limitations from an early age. Encouraging routines that include stretching, gentle strength training, and activities that promote body awareness can offer significant benefits in the future. Additionally, integrating assistive devices, such as supportive braces or specially designed backpacks, can alleviate stress on the spine during daily activities and prevent further complications.

Equally important is addressing the emotional impact of these adaptations. Teaching your child coping strategies through mindfulness practices can play a pivotal role in building resilience and self-confidence. Mindfulness practices such as guided meditations, mindful breathing exercises, and yoga can help your child become more aware of their body's needs and responses. These practices teach them to observe their discomfort without judgment, providing them with the skills to manage pain and stress in a healthy way.

Art therapy and participation in supportive community programs also contribute to emotional strength, offering creative outlets and peer support that emphasize they are not alone in their journey. By framing these adaptations as tools for enhancing quality of life rather than restrictions, you empower your child to take control of their scoliosis journey.

While more intense pain typically emerges in adulthood, the proactive steps taken now can pave the way for a healthier, more active future. By emphasizing that these adaptations are part of a broader strategy to manage scoliosis, you help your child understand that they can lead a full and rewarding life despite the challenges posed by the condition. This approach not only alleviates physical discomfort but also strengthens mental and emotional well-being, equipping your child with the tools they need to face their future with optimism and strength. This perspective fosters a proactive stance toward scoliosis management, focusing on improvement and regular monitoring rather than seeking an unattainable cure, thus setting a realistic and empowering path forward.

10. What to Expect if Scoliosis is not Addressed?

Ignoring scoliosis and hoping it will go away on its own is not a viable option. While it might seem tempting to think that the condition will fix itself over time, untreated scoliosis often leads to worsening symptoms and an increased risk of complications. One common misconception is that scoliosis stops progressing once the body reaches skeletal maturity. The reality is that scoliosis continues to progress, just at a much slower pace. It may advance by only half a degree or a full degree every few years, which might not seem like much at first. But over the course of 20 years, what initially appeared to be a mild curve can become a severe spinal deformity, affecting posture, mobility, and overall quality of life.

Skeletal maturity is measured using X-rays, specifically looking at the Risser sign, which evaluates the level of bone growth at the iliac crest (the top part of the pelvis). The Risser sign is a scale from 0 to 5, with 0 indicating no skeletal maturity and 5 indicating full maturity, meaning the growth plates have closed. Generally, girls reach skeletal maturity around ages 12 to 14, while boys tend to reach skeletal maturity a bit later, around ages 14 to 16.

Doctors often believe that once a child reaches skeletal maturity, the spine's growth slows significantly, and they predict that the curvature won't worsen as dramatically. This belief stems from the idea that once the bones stop growing, the spine will have less ability to curve further.

However, while this may slow down the progression, it doesn't necessarily stop it completely, especially if the curvature is severe or the spine is still under stress from compensatory movements. Without intervention, scoliosis can result in more pronounced deformities, leading to increased pain, stiffness, and discomfort as the body works harder to compensate for the imbalance.

Over time, this ongoing strain can cause degenerative changes in the spine, heightening the risk of complications such as spinal cord compression, nerve damage, and in severe cases, respiratory difficulties. These complications can affect the most basic functions like breathing and standing for prolonged periods.

This is why it's crucial to keep monitoring the condition, even after your child reaches skeletal maturity. While the progression may slow down, it can still worsen if left untreated. The earlier you act, the better your chances of slowing or even halting the progression. By managing scoliosis proactively, rather than waiting for it to become debilitating, you can help preserve spinal health, function, and quality of life over the long term. Just like any health condition, the more you invest in prevention and early treatment, the better the outcomes will be.

11. It's Never Going to Get Better on Its Own

The harsh reality is that scoliosis is a progressive condition that requires proactive management to prevent worsening symptoms and complications. While it may be tempting to ignore the problem and hope for the best, the truth is that scoliosis will not improve on its own. Without intervention, the curvature of the spine will continue to worsen over time, leading to increased pain, disability, and loss of function.

What starts as a mild curve in childhood can gradually progress into a debilitating condition in adulthood, affecting not only posture but also mobility, confidence, and overall quality of life. The body compensates for the imbalance, leading to chronic pain, muscle fatigue, and an increased risk of degenerative spinal conditions such as arthritis, disc herniations, and nerve compression.

In severe cases, scoliosis can impact lung function and internal organ health, making even simple activities like walking, standing, or breathing more difficult. It's important to understand that while regular exercise like gym workouts or yoga is beneficial for overall health, they do not specifically correct the imbalances caused by scoliosis. These activities will not harm individuals with scoliosis and are encouraged for their general health benefits, but scoliosis requires targeted, corrective exercises designed specifically to address the spinal curvature. These exercises are essential in realigning the spine, strengthening core muscles, and ensuring that the body maintains better posture.

The longer scoliosis is left unaddressed, the fewer treatment options remain. Waiting until the condition becomes unbearable often means resorting to invasive procedures like spinal fusion surgery, which comes with its own risks and permanent limitations. Early intervention is the key to maintaining spinal health, preventing long-term complications, and preserving an active, pain-free lifestyle. You wouldn't ignore a cavity and expect it to fix itself; scoliosis is no different. The best thing you can do for yourself, or your child is to act now before the condition dictates your future.

By understanding the progressive nature of scoliosis and recognizing that active, specific interventions are necessary, you can take informed steps to manage the condition effectively. This approach not only helps in alleviating immediate symptoms but also in preventing the progression of the curvature. Investing in a tailored exercise program and regular check-ups with a specialist who understands the complexities of scoliosis can make a significant difference in quality of life and long-term health outcomes.

Section 3: Can you do something about their scoliosis?

12. What Does Successful Treatment Looks Like?

Successful treatment for scoliosis is more than just managing symptoms, it's about reclaiming a life that isn't dictated by pain, discomfort, or self-consciousness. For some, success means being able to move freely without restriction, participate in activities they love, and go through their day without chronic pain weighing them down. For others, it's about improving posture, breathing more easily, and standing taller with confidence. True success isn't just measured by X-rays or degrees of curvature; it's about how they feel in their own body and how scoliosis impacts their daily life.

It's important to remember that not all successful outcomes are measured by X-ray results. I've had cases where everything improves, posture, performance, pain, strength, but the X-rays may not show significant change, and parents can feel discouraged, even cheated. In many cases, there are improvements in X-ray measurements, but there are instances where the changes are minimal or even nonexistent. This is why it's so crucial for parents to accept these outcomes without placing blame on the experts or, worse, on their children. If an expert fails to deliver the treatments they promised, then they can be held accountable, but remember, nothing in life is guaranteed. If an expert guarantees results, it's best to be cautious and stay away from them.

In my practice, I try to keep expectations realistic and conservative. Based on our past experiences and data, we estimate that a typical change in Cobb angle measurements from X-rays is around 5-8 degrees, assuming there is good compliance with the treatment plan. We can always tweak the program and adjust their results based on posture checks and Scoliometer readings.

Our spinal correction average, across all my experts and myself, tends to fall between 12-14 degrees, but I never promise that. It's better to expect less and be pleasantly surprised by greater results than to set unrealistic expectations and face disappointment.

Beyond physical improvements, successful treatment also brings emotional healing. Many individuals with scoliosis struggle with self-esteem issues due to visible changes in their posture, and this can take a toll on their confidence. The right treatment plan can help them regain control, not just over their spine, but over their mindset allowing them to feel strong, empowered, and capable. Ultimately, successful treatment means they are no longer defined by scoliosis; instead, they are actively shaping their own health and future.

13. Getting on the Same Page with People Who Can Help

Scoliosis treatment is not a solo journey it requires a dedicated support system, including healthcare providers, family members, and even friends who understand the challenges involved. The key to a successful treatment path is clear and open communication with everyone involved in the process. This means expressing concerns, asking questions, and ensuring that everyone, family and healthcare team, is aligned and working toward the same goals.

One of the most important aspects of this journey is building a relationship with the healthcare professionals you choose to help your child. I cannot stress enough how essential it is to get to know the team working with your child understanding their expertise, techniques, and expected outcomes. It's crucial to understand their approach and respect their professional judgment, especially when dealing with something as complex as scoliosis.

Many times, parents come to me expressing concerns about the techniques I use, often based on their previous experiences or research. While I genuinely appreciate the dedication, they have in wanting to improve their child's scoliosis, sometimes this can get in the way of implementing the recommended treatment plan. After seeing multiple specialists, undergoing various rounds of treatment, and conducting their own research, it's only natural to want to be as involved as possible. But at this point in the journey, trust becomes crucial. By the time parents bring their child to my team, they've often been through a long, winding path.

Once you've found the expert who you feel is the right fit for your child, trust them and allow them to perform the treatment that they believe will work best. Scoliosis treatment is never a quick fix or a one-size-fits-all approach, it's a journey, and the path will not be linear. There will be ups and downs, successes and setbacks.

Communication is vital throughout the process. It's essential to discuss any concerns and keep an open dialogue with your healthcare team but also respect their expertise in providing treatment.

The best experts are those who understand scoliosis as it is, a complex, multifactorial condition that requires a multidisciplinary approach. It's not just about applying one technique or method; it's about integrating various disciplines and techniques, each tailored to address different aspects of the condition.

By working with a team that uses a combination of approaches, your child has the best chance of achieving meaningful results.

In the end, a successful scoliosis treatment journey is one built on trust, communication, and a collaborative effort between the family and the healthcare professionals.

Dr. Juan Jesus Villa

With the right team, the right approach, and a solid support system, you can ensure that your child is receiving the best care possible.

14. Are Your Providers Specialized in Scoliosis?

Not all medical professionals have the expertise required to effectively manage scoliosis. A general healthcare provider may recognize the signs of scoliosis, but that doesn't mean they are equipped to treat it properly. When searching for care, it's essential to seek out specialists who have experience and training specifically in scoliosis management.

Scoliosis is a complex condition that requires specialized care, and the best outcomes often come from healthcare providers who focus on spinal deformities. Whether it's an orthopedic surgeon specializing in spinal deformities, a chiropractor trained in scoliosis-specific rehabilitation, or a physical therapist skilled in targeted exercises, these specialists are the ones who truly understand the intricacies of scoliosis and can offer personalized treatment plans that go far beyond generic advice. They stay up to date on the latest advancements in both non-surgical and surgical interventions, helping families make informed, confident decisions about the care their child will receive.

When looking for a scoliosis specialist, certifications might seem like an obvious place to start. They often signify formal training and knowledge in a specific area. However, I have seen many cases where a specialist's credentials or certifications were not enough to deliver the results patients were hoping for. The sad truth is that certifications are often used as marketing tools to promote a professional or attract more clients. I've even had to send patients to other professionals who had impressive credentials or who had attended well-known seminars, only to be disappointed by the methods and outcomes.

I've always believed that true expertise comes from continuous learning, not from accumulating certificates. Throughout my career, I've taken many advanced courses to expand my knowledge and improve the care I provide. My focus has never been on collecting titles or paying for listings on websites, but on genuinely understanding the methods that deliver the best results for my patients.

Experience is the true measure of a provider's skill. Don't just focus on what certifications they hold, look at their history of successful cases, the techniques they use, and their approach to treatment. It's just as important, if not more so, to ask about their not-so-successful cases. No provider has a 100% success rate, it's simply not possible. A trustworthy provider will be open about the challenges they've faced, with real-life examples that show what worked, what didn't, and most importantly, why. Transparency and honesty in a provider's track record can help you determine if they are the right fit for you or your child.

Choosing the right provider isn't about credentials alone, it's about finding someone who listens, understands, and creates a treatment plan tailored to your child's unique needs. The wrong provider can lead to mismanagement, unnecessary delays, and frustration, while the right one can make all the difference in avoiding future pain and complications, giving your child the best chance at a healthier, more active future.

15. A Picture of What's Possible

One of the most powerful motivators in scoliosis treatment is seeing what's possible. When you first start your child's scoliosis treatment journey, it's easy to feel uncertain about the future, wondering if they will ever live a pain-free life, have the freedom to move without discomfort, or be able to fully enjoy activities they love. But as you witness others who have successfully navigated the same path, it can become incredibly motivating. These stories are a reminder that improvement is not just a distant hope, it is possible with the right approach.

Before-and-after images, personal testimonies, and success stories serve as a tangible representation of progress. Many individuals, children included, have transformed their lives through a carefully chosen combination of treatments, whether it's bracing, physical therapy, or, in some cases, surgery. These real-life examples show that, with dedication, patience, and proper guidance, scoliosis can be managed effectively, and improvement is absolutely within reach. It's important to remember that even small improvements can make a significant difference in the quality of life, and these changes build up over time.

A future with better posture, reduced pain, and a more fulfilling life isn't just a dream it's a reality for those who commit to the process. The key is to start now and take control of scoliosis before it progresses further. It's about consistently acting, even when the results aren't immediately visible. Progress in scoliosis treatment is often gradual, with setbacks along the way, but those setbacks don't mean failure, they simply mean that the path is not always linear.

Trust the process, remain consistent, and believe that positive change is not only possible, but highly achievable. With the right support from healthcare providers, family, and a community who understands the challenges, you and your child can reclaim health, confidence, and a brighter future. While the road may be long, with the right mindset and dedication, there is so much hope for a better, pain-free tomorrow. Keep going and know that every step forward counts.

Section 4: Should Your Child Have Scoliosis Surgery?

16. What Is It Like to Have Spinal Fusion Surgery for Scoliosis?

Spinal fusion surgery is a significant and invasive procedure that is often recommended for severe cases of scoliosis. It is typically considered when the curvature of the spine reaches a certain degree, often around 40 to 50 degrees, though this can vary depending on the severity and the age of the patient. Surgeons may also consider surgery if the curve is causing significant pain, mobility issues, or complications such as nerve compression. In some cases, if the curvature is progressive and seems likely to worsen, surgery may be recommended even if the curve hasn't yet reached the critical threshold.

During the operation, the surgeon works to straighten the spine as much as possible and secures it with metal rods, screws, or other stabilizing devices. Bone grafts, materials designed to encourage bone healing and regeneration, are placed along the curved areas of the spine. Over time, these grafts fuse with the surrounding vertebrae, creating a solid, immobile structure that helps prevent further curvature.

While spinal fusion can provide significant relief and stop the curve from progressing, it is important to understand that this procedure is not a quick fix, nor is it without risks.

The recovery process after spinal fusion is long, challenging, and often painful. Since the spine is essentially made immobile, the body must adjust to its new structure. The initial recovery period involves considerable pain and discomfort. Many patients experience restricted movement, and simple activities like bending, sitting for long periods, or even getting out of bed may be difficult for a while.

The loss of spinal mobility is one of the most significant challenges after surgery, as the fusion prevents the spine from moving as it once did. This can lead to stiffness and limitations in flexibility, which can be frustrating, especially for individuals who were previously active.

In some cases, even after spinal fusion, scoliosis can start to reappear elsewhere in the body as a compensatory mechanism. Since the spine is no longer mobile, the rest of the body may adjust by shifting alignment in other areas, which can lead to pain or discomfort in new regions.

This is why rehabilitation after surgery is crucial. The process of rehabilitation and physical therapy helps retrain the body to move properly, realign the muscles, and correct any imbalances caused by the lack of movement in the fused spine. Physical therapy is just as important after surgery as it was before, as it helps the body adjust to the structural changes and prevents new issues from arising.

If you are considering surgery, it should be because you have tried alternative treatments first, and surgery is the best approach for your child's unique situation. Surgery should rarely be the first option unless necessary, and it's important to exhaust other options such as bracing, physical therapy, and rehabilitation before making this decision.

Remember, even after surgery, the need for rehabilitation doesn't go away. In fact, the body needs to be retrained to function in this new way. Your child's recovery doesn't end once they leave the operating room rehabilitation is essential for building strength, flexibility, and long-term function.

While spinal fusion can be life-changing in a positive way, it's crucial to recognize that this is a journey, one that requires careful consideration, ongoing support, and a realistic understanding of what recovery entails.

It's not a "quick fix," but it can offer lasting results for those with severe scoliosis, providing relief from pain, halting progression of the curve, and improving long-term quality of life. However, it's essential to have realistic expectations about the recovery process, the challenges that come with it, and the need for long-term care and rehabilitation.

17. Surgery Creates a New Normal: What Will That Mean for Them?

One of the most profound challenges after spinal fusion surgery is adjusting to life with a spine that no longer moves the way it once did. The fused segments create a permanent stiffness, limiting flexibility and restricting certain movements that were once second nature.

Simple activities like bending over to tie a shoe, twisting to look behind, or engaging in sports that require agility can become difficult or even impossible. Many patients describe a constant awareness of their spine feeling rigid, and some experience chronic discomfort due to the altered biomechanics of their body.

This loss of mobility can be frustrating, especially for young individuals who were once active and unrestricted in their movement. Over time, other areas of the spine may compensate for the lack of motion, leading to added stress and potential pain in adjacent segments.

However, if surgery was the decision you made for your child, or if surgery has already happened without fully realizing all available options, please don't feel guilty or regretful. Many families come to this decision because it seemed like the best option at the time, and that's okay. Every decision in scoliosis treatment should be made based on what seems right for that child and their circumstances, with the knowledge available at that time.

No decision should be clouded with guilt; instead, recognize that, in the moment, it was likely the best option for your child's health and well-being. You're doing the best you can for your child, and that's what truly matters.

Beyond the physical adjustments, the emotional journey after surgery can be just as significant. Many individuals feel relief that their scoliosis has been stabilized, but some struggle with the reality that their body no longer moves the way it once did.

Frustration, disappointment, or even grief over lost mobility can be part of the process. It's important to recognize that adjusting to a fused spine takes time both mentally and physically. Some may feel different or even less "whole" because of the physical changes to their body, such as the presence of scars, altered posture, or restricted movement. For teenagers, in particular, the adjustment can be difficult, as they are already navigating a time of self-consciousness and body changes. The reality of adjusting to a "new normal" may be overwhelming for them at first.

As a mother, this is where your role becomes so crucial. Be patient with your child as they adapt to this new chapter in their life. Their physical changes, including visible scars, may be a source of discomfort or self-consciousness. Their mobility will change, and they may struggle with activities they once enjoyed. Sports, for example, may no longer feel the same, and they might experience feelings of loss or frustration.

It's important to encourage them through this period of transition. Remind them that it's okay to take time to adjust and that this is just a new phase of their journey. Let them know that their self-worth is not tied to how much they can move or how they look but to their strength, resilience, and character.

Even after surgery, your child still needs to retrain their body and mind. Rehabilitation is a crucial part of their recovery, as it helps them regain strength and improve their mobility within the limits of their fused spine. It's important to support them through the physical challenges of rehabilitation, and to be empathetic when they express emotional frustration or sadness about their "new normal." This may be a time for you as a family to lean into support groups, therapy, or other resources that can help both you and your child process these changes.

With patience, support, and the right rehabilitation, individuals can find ways to adapt to their new body and continue leading fulfilling lives. The emotional toll of these limitations can be just as challenging as the physical recovery, making it crucial for families to fully understand the long-term impact of spinal fusion before deciding.

However, it's equally important to know that, with time, your child will likely find a new rhythm, and while things may never be quite the same, they can still lead an active and healthy life. They will adapt, and so will you. This is a journey that requires time, love, and understanding, but with your ongoing support, they can rise above the challenges and embrace their "new normal."

18. Surgery Isn't the End of Scoliosis

Many people assume that once spinal fusion surgery is complete, scoliosis is "fixed." While spinal fusion can provide significant improvement, it is not a cure, it's a structural correction, and it comes with lifelong considerations. The surgery itself addresses the curvature in a major way, but it's important to understand that scoliosis is a dynamic condition, meaning that the spine will continue to evolve over time, even after surgery.

Recovery is just the beginning of this journey, and ongoing care is essential to maintaining spinal health in the long term. Even after the surgery, regular monitoring is still crucial. Just because the spine has been fused doesn't mean the scoliosis won't progress in other parts of the spine or elsewhere in the body. Over time, the body may begin to compensate for the fused segments, and those compensatory changes can lead to new issues or discomfort.

This is why monitoring remains a key part of the post-surgical process, much like any other treatment plan. The best approach is to treat it as if the child were still undergoing other treatments and to remain proactive in monitoring their spinal health.

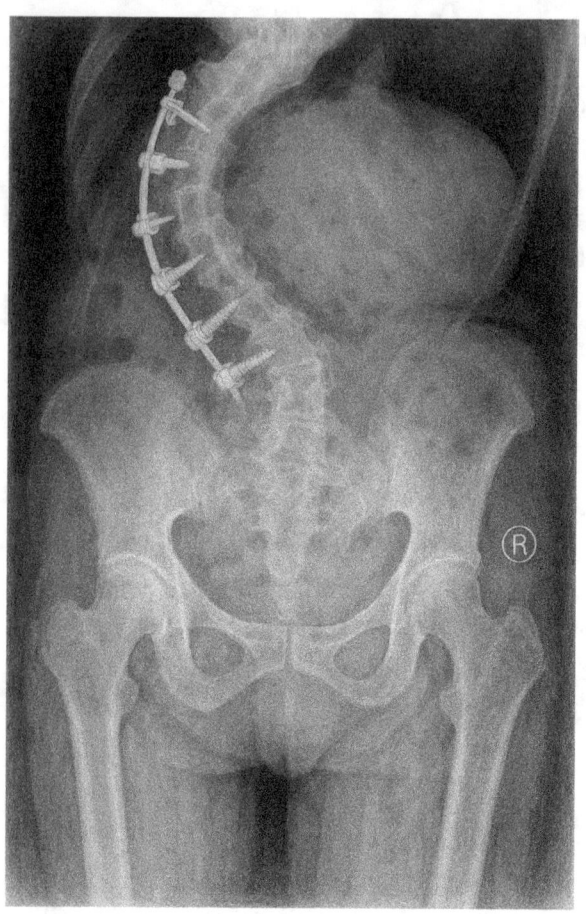

This is an artistic representation of one of my own patients. A 68 female with spinal fusion done at age 20. You can see how the spine still worsened years after surgery.

Follow-up appointments, regular X-rays to track changes, rehabilitation exercises, and posture checks should continue even after surgery. You might notice that the spine feels different, and the body is adjusting to a new way of moving. Keep encouraging your child to stay active, but within their limitations. Even with surgery, it's vital to maintain physical activity to prevent stiffness and keep the muscles strong.

At the same time, watch for signs of overcompensation in the body, whether it's poor posture or new areas of pain, and address them early. Compensating for the immobile spine can lead to strain on other parts of the body, so remaining vigilant and adjusting is important.

Regular chiropractic care is highly recommended after surgery to help your child adapt to their "new normal." Chiropractic care, particularly post-surgical rehabilitation, can help address these compensations and support proper spinal alignment.

Chiropractors who specialize in scoliosis understand the biomechanics of a fused spine and can provide tailored adjustments to ensure that the body adapts properly to the changes, preventing undue stress on the rest of the spine and the body as a whole. With consistent chiropractic care, the body can better compensate for the lack of movement in the fused segments, helping to minimize discomfort and improve overall mobility.

It's also important to remember that spinal fusion surgery does not prevent degeneration in other parts of the spine. The unfused sections of the spine can still experience increased strain over time, potentially leading to new issues, such as arthritis, disc degeneration, or even pain in the surrounding areas. This is why post-surgical care is just as important as the surgery itself. Staying active, following medical advice, attending regular check-ups, and prioritizing spinal health will all contribute to long-term well-being.

Ultimately, spinal fusion surgery can help provide stability and relieve symptoms of scoliosis. It's a process that doesn't stop after the surgery. It's essential to continue monitoring, adjusting, and supporting your child as they grow and adapt to their new body. With the right ongoing care and attention, they can still lead a fulfilling, active life. Encourage your child to embrace their new normal and support them through the ongoing journey of maintaining their spinal health.

19. Surgery Is No Longer the Gold Standard for Scoliosis Treatment

For many years, spinal fusion surgery was considered the gold standard for scoliosis treatment, especially in severe cases. It was often seen as the final solution when the curve became too pronounced or began to cause debilitating pain or loss of function. However, over the years, significant advancements in non-surgical treatments have shifted this perspective.

Today, families have more choices than ever before. Conservative approaches such as bracing, scoliosis-specific chiropractic care, targeted exercises, and physical therapy are increasingly recognized as effective alternatives that can prevent the progression of the curve and, in some cases, even reduce the severity of scoliosis.

These non-surgical treatments are particularly beneficial for children and adolescents, whose spines are still growing and are therefore more responsive to intervention. By utilizing therapies that focus on spinal alignment, strengthening muscles, and improving posture, many children can avoid the need for surgery altogether. Even in adults, specialized programs in chiropractic care, physical therapy, and rehabilitation can yield substantial improvements, from pain relief to enhanced mobility and functionality.

Dr. Juan Jesus Villa

The goal is to stabilize the spine, reduce discomfort, and maintain an active lifestyle without resorting to invasive procedures unless necessary.

Surgical techniques have evolved over time, with newer, less invasive options offering better outcomes and shorter recovery periods. However, it's important to note that even with these advancements, surgery still carries risks, and once performed, it is irreversible. This has led many families to explore conservative treatments before jumping to surgery. With the growing success of non-surgical methods, surgery is no longer the automatic next step, it has become one option among many. In fact, for many patients, surgery may not be necessary at all. This shift in thinking reflects the growing body of evidence supporting the effectiveness of holistic, multi-disciplinary treatment plans that focus on long-term spine health, not just short-term corrections.

If you're considering treatment options for your child's scoliosis, it's crucial to know that you have options. It's understandable to feel pressure or anxiety, especially when faced with a diagnosis, but rushing into surgery out of fear or a sense of urgency is not the only path forward. Educate yourself about all available treatments, including non-surgical methods that could help slow the progression of the curve, improve posture, and reduce pain. Many parents feel a sense of relief knowing that surgery doesn't have to be the first step, and they can explore less invasive treatments that might provide the results they're hoping for.

I often work with families who initially considered surgery as their only option, but after exploring alternative treatments, such as scoliosis-specific chiropractic care and physical therapy, they realize that surgery might not be necessary after all. It's not about denying the option of surgery when it is truly needed, but rather about giving families the opportunity to explore other methods first and make informed decisions. Remember, scoliosis treatment is not a "one size fits all." The right choice for your child is the one that considers their individual needs, their stage of growth, and their overall well-being.

When you take a step back and explore all available treatments, you're not only empowering yourself as a parent but you're also giving your child the best chance to improve their quality of life while avoiding unnecessary procedures.

The right decision prioritizes both spinal health and overall quality of life, helping to shape a future where your child can live pain-free, confident, and active. This shift in treatment philosophy offers hope for families, giving them the tools to make the best decisions for their child and their future health.

Section 5: Effective Scoliosis Treatment

20. Scoliosis-Specific Chiropractic

As a parent, it's natural to want the best for your child, especially when it comes to their health. A scoliosis diagnosis can be overwhelming and often comes with a sense of urgency. You may feel uncertain about the best path forward, but rest assured, there are treatment options that can help manage your child's condition effectively. One such option is scoliosis-specific chiropractic care, a highly specialized approach that is designed to address the unique spinal imbalances and structural distortions associated with scoliosis.

Unlike traditional chiropractic care, which typically focuses on relieving misalignments in the spine through standard adjustments, scoliosis-specific chiropractic care goes far beyond that. This type of chiropractic integrates a combination of specialized spinal corrections, traction therapies, neuromuscular retraining, and rehabilitative exercises.

These techniques work synergistically to influence spinal alignment, improve posture, and reduce excessive strain on the muscles and ligaments that support the spine. By addressing the root causes of the spinal curvature, scoliosis-specific chiropractic care aims to improve both function and comfort for your child.

One of the key differences between conventional chiropractic care and scoliosis-specific chiropractic is the understanding that scoliosis is a three-dimensional condition. The curvature is not just a simple bend in the spine, but a complex, dynamic issue that affects the spine in multiple planes: side-to-side, back-to-front, and rotationally.

This is why scoliosis requires a precise, customized treatment approach, rather than a "one-size-fits-all" method. Traditional chiropractic techniques, while helpful for general spinal health, don't address the unique complexities of scoliosis, making specialized chiropractic care necessary for effective treatment.

Scoliosis-specific chiropractic focuses on correcting the underlying biomechanical dysfunction that contributes to the curvature. By making targeted adjustments, chiropractors aim to slow, halt, or even reverse the progression of the curve.

In many cases, this approach can reduce discomfort, improve mobility, and help restore functional movement. It's important to note that scoliosis-specific chiropractic care doesn't simply aim to treat symptoms; it addresses the root causes of scoliosis, focusing on long-term spinal health and stability.

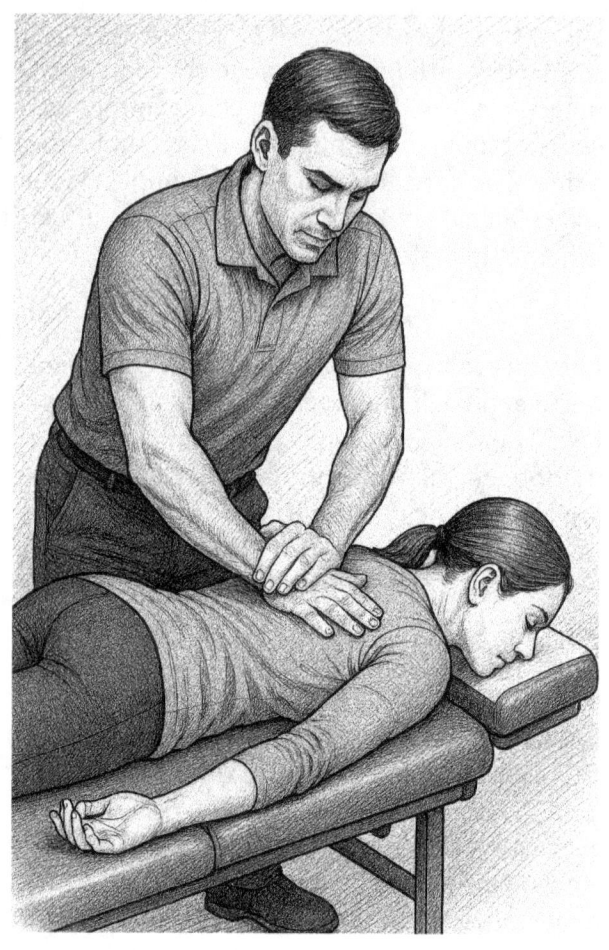

This illustration demonstrates a chiropractic adjustment on the scoliotic segments.

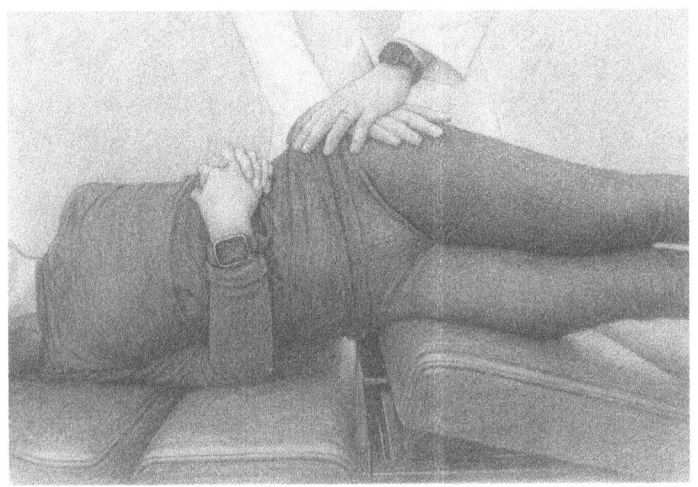

Demonstration of scoliosis specific chiropractic adjustment.

Another significant advantage of scoliosis-specific chiropractic is that it is non-invasive. Unlike surgery or medication, chiropractic care does not involve any cutting or drugs. It is a natural approach that works with the body's own mechanics to promote healing and proper alignment.

Moreover, scoliosis-specific chiropractic care doesn't rely on a "wait-and-see" approach. Many traditional treatments, like simply monitoring the curve over time, allow the condition to worsen gradually without intervention. Instead, scoliosis-specific chiropractic actively works to slow or even reverse the progression of the curvature, offering a proactive way to manage scoliosis before it becomes more debilitating.

In addition to spinal adjustments, many chiropractic treatments incorporate traction therapies, which are designed to gently elongate the spine. This helps to reduce the compressive forces on the spine and facilitates the realignment of the vertebrae.

Spinal rehabilitation focuses on strengthening and re-educating the muscles that support the spine, helping to improve posture and reduce muscle imbalances. Rehabilitative exercises are also used to ensure that the muscles remain balanced and functional, allowing for improved mobility and strength. This multi-modal approach ensures that all aspects of scoliosis are addressed, including the muscles, joints, and overall alignment.

Importantly, scoliosis-specific chiropractic care is not just about managing pain; it's about restoring functionality and improving quality of life. It's an active process that requires commitment and consistency. As your child's spine undergoes treatment, it's essential to stay engaged with the process. Regular check-ups, monitoring progress, and following through with prescribed exercises and adjustments are crucial for long-term success.

Many parents choose scoliosis-specific chiropractic care because it offers a non-invasive, personalized treatment option that not only addresses the curvature but also strengthens the body as a whole. It gives children the best possible chance to maintain a strong, healthy spine while avoiding the need for invasive treatments, such as surgery. This approach actively works to improve the condition rather than simply waiting for things to worsen.

Scoliosis-specific chiropractic care works by understanding the complexity of scoliosis and using a combination of targeted techniques to address it. It is a holistic, non-invasive treatment method that focuses on long-term spinal health, improved posture, and reduced discomfort. By addressing scoliosis early and taking a proactive approach, you are helping your child not only manage their condition but also improve their overall quality of life.

21. Understanding Spinal Traction in Scoliosis Management

In the treatment of scoliosis, spinal traction is a cornerstone therapeutic approach used in many clinics to address the complex dynamics of spinal deformities. Two primary forms of spinal traction are employed: decompression traction and structural traction, each serving distinct but complementary roles in scoliosis treatment.

Decompression Traction

Decompression traction is a technique designed to alleviate pressure on the spine while promoting vertical elongation, or expansion along the y-axis. This form of traction effectively counteracts the compressive forces of gravity on the spinal column, facilitating the unwinding process in the spinal alignment. As the spine elongates, space is created between the vertebrae, which can lead to significant relief from back pain and discomfort associated with scoliosis. The real power of decompression traction lies in its ability to be combined with corrective exercises. When used together, these therapies can encourage the spine to adopt a more natural alignment, gradually improving the curvature characteristic of scoliosis. The spine's ability to unwind and straighten is enhanced, making this approach a vital part of a comprehensive scoliosis management plan.

Structural Traction

On the other hand, structural traction focuses on bending the spine towards a corrective posture. Originally developed by practitioners of Chiropractic Biophysics, this method aims to stretch and elongate the spinal ligaments, allowing for physical remodeling of the spine's structure. Structural traction is designed to address the lateral or side-to-side curvature of the spine by applying a consistent force to mold the spine into a more typical alignment.

Clinical studies support the efficacy of structural traction, demonstrating that long-term biomechanical adaptation requires sustained force over extended periods. The traction must be applied consistently to achieve and maintain correction of spinal postural distortions. After approximately 10 minutes of continuous traction, the spinal ligaments begin to stretch sufficiently to enable true structural changes. This duration is crucial as it crosses the threshold beyond which permanent, corrective alterations in the ligament structure can begin to take root.

Both types of traction underscore the necessity of time and consistency in the treatment of scoliosis. Regular and prolonged application of traction forces is essential for making lasting changes to the spine's posture. The effectiveness of traction therapy is not just in the force applied but in how consistency and duration.

Dr. Juan Jesus Villa

Patients undergoing traction therapy must commit to regular sessions over an extended period to see significant improvements in their spinal curvature and overall posture.

Traction therapy offers a promising non-surgical option for many individuals living with scoliosis. By understanding and utilizing both decompression and structural traction techniques, practitioners can provide targeted treatments that address the specific needs and conditions of their patients.

For those with scoliosis, these traction therapies represent hope for not only stopping progression but also potentially reversing some of the adverse effects of this complex spinal condition.

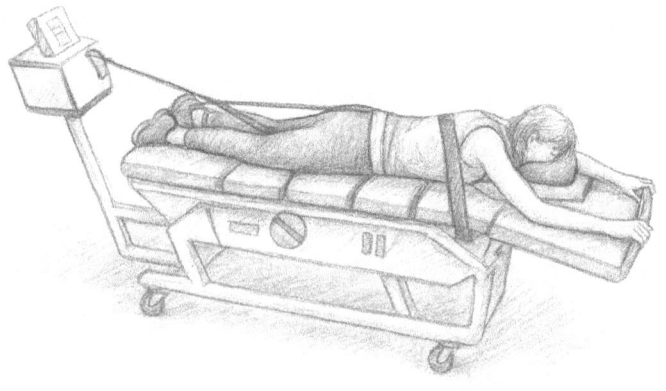

Decompression traction designed to elongate the spine enabling scoliosis correction.

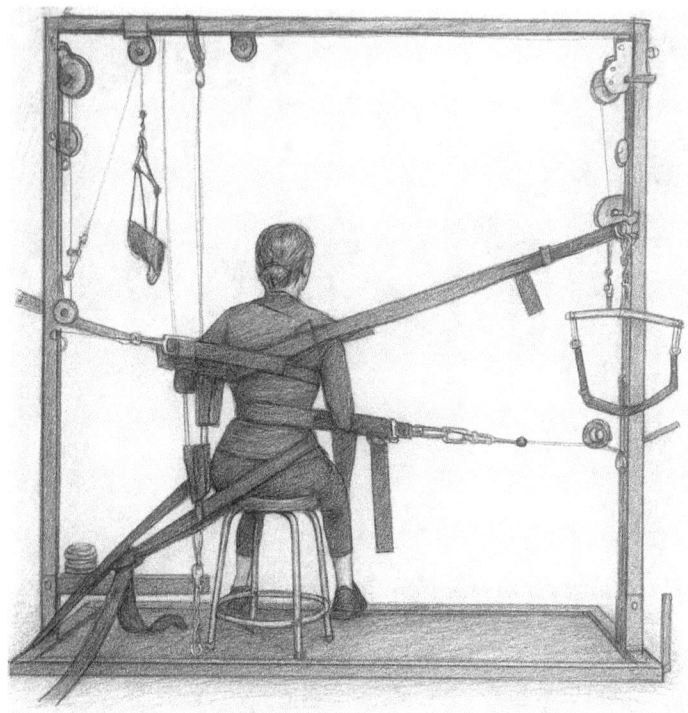

Structural traction provides sideways traction force to unbend the scoliotic curvature.

22. Scoliosis-Bracing

The thought of your child needing a scoliosis brace can be overwhelming. It's not just a medical device it's a constant, visible reminder of the condition your child is facing, and for many children, it symbolizes the uncertainty and challenges that come with scoliosis. Bracing is often prescribed to slow the progression of spinal curvature during growth, applying gentle but consistent pressure to guide the spine into a more stable position. However, it's important to understand that a brace is not a cure and will not fix scoliosis on its own. Rather, it is a tool, a critical part of a comprehensive treatment plan that includes scoliosis-specific chiropractic care, physical therapy, and corrective exercises.

Bracing can certainly be effective when used alongside these other treatments, but many parents mistakenly believe that just wearing the brace will automatically correct the curvature. This is not the case. While braces can help reduce the curvature, their effectiveness depends on their use as part of an overall strategy to improve spinal health, function, and posture. It's crucial that the brace is seen as part of the process, not the entire solution.

The experience of wearing a brace can be both physically and emotionally challenging for your child. The initial discomfort, self-consciousness, and sense of restriction can make this process difficult, and as a mother, it's heartbreaking to watch your child struggle with these adjustments. However, the good news is that there are different types of braces, each designed to serve specific needs and address different areas of scoliosis. Understanding these options can help you make an informed decision and choose the best one for your child's unique situation.

There are several types of braces commonly used for scoliosis. The Boston Brace is one of the most used braces for scoliosis, and it is a rigid plastic shell that fits around the trunk, worn under clothing. It's designed for thoracic and lumbar curves, typically for children with curves in the lower and mid-back regions. The Boston brace applies consistent pressure to the spine, helping to prevent further progression of the curve during growth. Although it can be uncomfortable and restrictive, it is effective at slowing or halting curve progression if worn consistently.

The Milwaukee Brace is a more extensive option, extending from the pelvis to the neck. It is typically used for higher thoracic curves, especially those that affect the upper spine. The Milwaukee brace is designed to apply corrective force to the upper spine and ribs and is generally worn under clothing, but its bulk can be challenging for children to adjust to, especially when it comes to comfort and body image. While it can be effective, the emotional toll can be considerable, so it's essential to provide your child with consistent emotional support during treatment.

The Charleston Bending Brace is designed to be worn at night and offers a more flexible option for children who need to wear a brace for long periods. The Charleston Bending Brace allows for greater freedom during the day, providing more comfort while still helping to correct the curvature.

The design targets specific curvatures by gently bending the spine in the opposite direction, providing corrective pressure while your child sleeps. For some children, this option works well because it allows them to be more active during the day.

The Dynamic Brace is often favored by both children and parents because it allows greater flexibility and movement compared to more rigid braces. It doesn't immobilize the spine but instead works with the body to encourage better alignment and support while allowing muscles to remain active. This is important because when the spine is held in place for too long without movement, the muscles can weaken and become dependent on the brace.

The Dynamic Brace encourages proper posture and muscle engagement, which can be beneficial for overall spinal health. It also permits your child to engage in light sports, walking, and bending, making it a more tolerable option for daily life. However, even with its flexibility, it is still important to remember that bracing alone is not a cure. It must be combined with other therapeutic interventions like chiropractic care and physical therapy, to be truly effective.

No matter which brace is chosen, it is crucial to remember that a brace is not a standalone solution. It's a tool to aid therapy, not a replacement for comprehensive treatment. Even though a brace helps to prevent further progression of the curve, it does not address the underlying imbalances in the body that cause scoliosis in the first place. Without proper exercise, chiropractic care, and a targeted rehabilitation plan, bracing can only go so far in managing scoliosis.

This brings us to the emotional and social aspect of bracing. It's important to understand that wearing a brace is not just a physical treatment, it can also have a significant impact on your child's self-esteem and social life. Bracing can be a source of embarrassment for some children, especially if the brace is visible or makes them feel different from their peers.

Many children experience self-consciousness and isolation due to the visibility of the brace. As a mother, it's essential to acknowledge these emotional challenges and support your child through this process. Encourage open conversations about their feelings and help them focus on the positive aspects of the treatment, such as how it will ultimately help them maintain better health and avoid surgery.

Moreover, it's important for parents to remember that bracing is most effective when it's part of a comprehensive treatment plan that includes scoliosis-specific chiropractic care, physical therapy, and corrective exercises. Bracing, along with these other methods, can significantly improve the quality of life and spinal function for your child, allowing them to continue leading a relatively active and pain-free life.

Choosing the right brace for your child is an important decision, but it's also vital to understand that bracing should never be seen as the complete solution. It is a tool that helps your child maintain the best possible spinal health, and when used in conjunction with other therapies, it can be very effective. Encourage your child to stay active, continue with their exercises, and work closely with their healthcare providers.

Remember, the brace is only part of the treatment plan. It's about empowering your child to continue their journey toward better health while supporting them emotionally through the process. The goal is not just to stop the progression of the curve, but to promote overall spinal health, help your child feel more confident, and provide them with the tools they need to adapt to the challenges of scoliosis with strength and resilience.

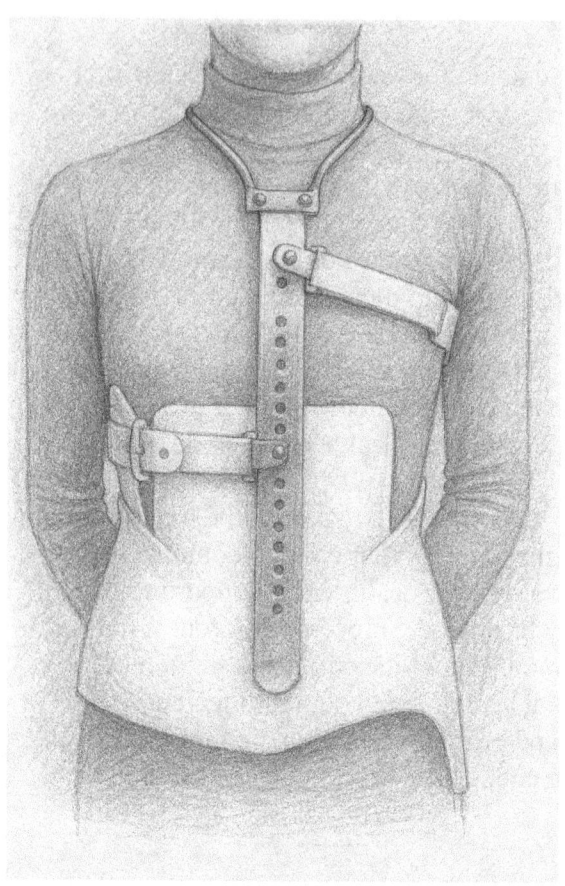

Illustration of the Milwaukee Brace. The rod extending to the neck region is designed to improve upper thoracic (upper back) scoliosis.

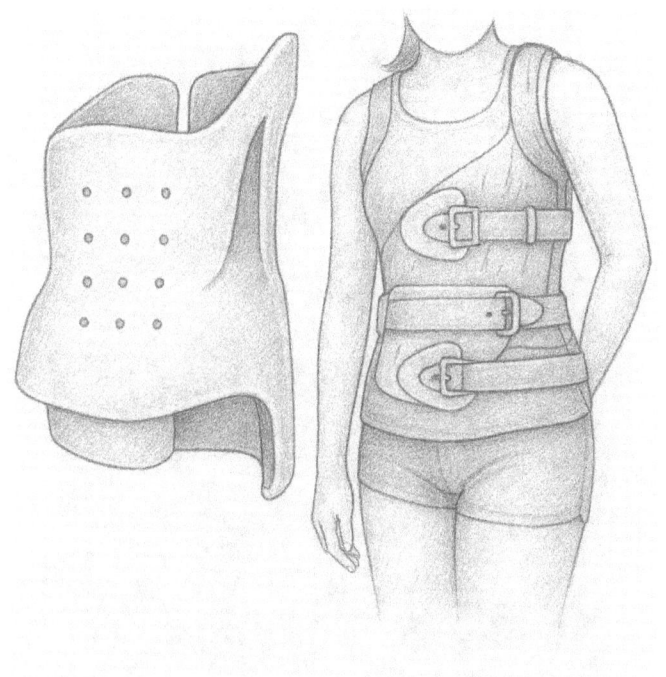

Left figure is the Boston Brace. The Boston Brace is one of the most recommended braces by specialists. The child will be instructed to wear it for 20-22 hours. The right figure is the Charleston Brace. Charleston Brace is recommended more for smaller scoliosis and only suggested to be used for sleeping.

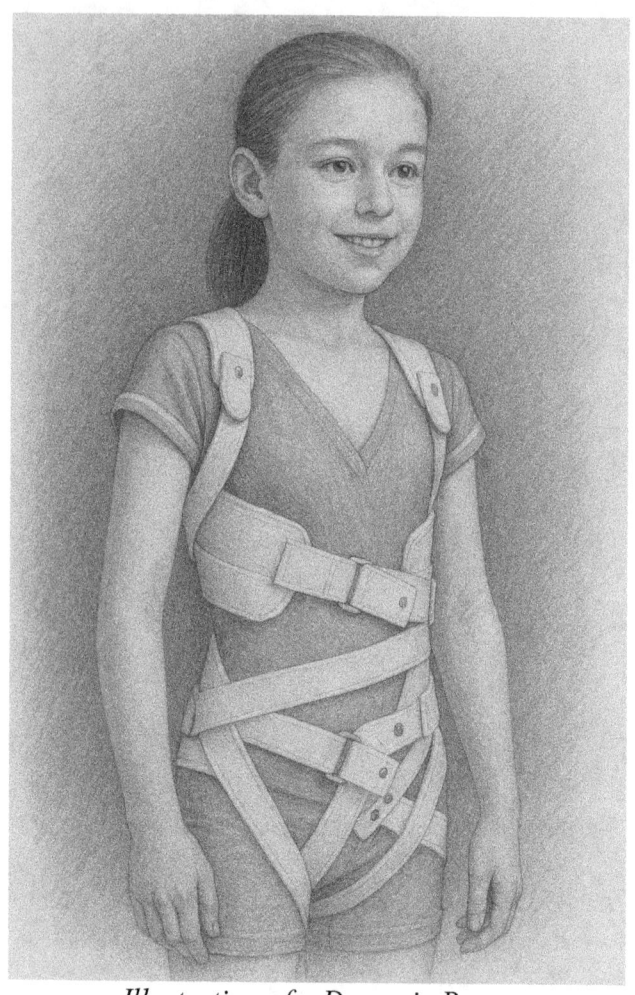

*Illustration of a Dynamic Brace
(flexible brace). For scoliosis that are not severe and
the child is willing to do more corrective exercises or
participate in sport themselves a dynamic brace is
recommend.*

23. What Results to Expect from Treatment?

It's natural to wonder: Will this treatment really help my child? While every scoliosis case is unique, many children experience noticeable improvements in posture, flexibility, and overall comfort with consistent care. In some cases, treatment can even reduce the severity of the curve, prevent future complications and reduce the likelihood of needing surgery. However, it's important to set realistic expectations and understand that each child's progress will vary.

The results of scoliosis treatment depend on several factors, including the severity of the curve, your child's age, and how closely the treatment plan is followed. Younger children, whose spines are still growing, tend to respond particularly well to early intervention. However, even if your child is older or has been living with scoliosis for some time, it's never too late to see improvement.

Many parents report that after starting scoliosis-specific chiropractic care, their child experiences less pain, better balance, and increased confidence in their movement. Additionally, improvements in strength and muscle tone are common, as the body adapts to better posture and proper alignment.

One of the key results parents often notice is an improvement in posture. With corrective exercises and chiropractic adjustments, the spine becomes better aligned, which can make a noticeable difference in how your child stands and moves. Not only does this help with the physical aspect of scoliosis, but it can also lead to improvements in their self-esteem. As they begin to stand taller and more confidently, many children experience a boost in their self-image and feel less self-conscious about their condition.

While complete curve correction isn't always possible, consistent care can make a significant difference in your child's health and daily life. X-ray measurements may show a reduction in the Cobb angle, but even if the changes are small, the improvements in your child's day-to-day functioning are what matter most. This might mean less pain, better range of motion, and the ability to participate in activities without feeling discomfort.

Some children even report that they experience less stiffness and do things they couldn't before, whether it's playing sports, engaging in physical activities, or simply being more active in everyday life.

It's essential to understand that the true measure of success is not just in the X-ray results, but in the overall improvements your child experiences in their daily life. While some may feel discouraged if they don't see drastic X-ray changes immediately, it's important to recognize that scoliosis treatment impacts far more than just the curve of the spine.

The emotional and physical benefits of better posture, less pain, and improved self-esteem are equally important and can have a lasting impact on your child's well-being.

In addition to physical improvements, treatment can also help your child develop better body mechanics. With regular adjustments and corrective exercises, your child will learn how to support their spine and maintain better posture throughout the day. This can help prevent further issues as they grow older and maintain a healthier spine.

The emotional benefits of treatment can also be profound. As your child feels better physically and gains confidence in their movement and posture, their self-esteem can improve significantly. Scoliosis can take a toll on a child's emotional well-being, but as they see progress and experience less discomfort, they may feel empowered to take control of their health and live more confidently.

The key to seeing these results is commitment, following through with prescribed exercises, attending regular chiropractic sessions, and making small lifestyle changes can all contribute to long-term success. Managing scoliosis is a journey, not a quick fix, and consistency is crucial. With patience, dedication, and the right treatment plan, your child has the potential to experience significant improvements in posture, strength, pain levels, and overall well-being. Remember, scoliosis treatment is not just about X-ray measurements, it's about improving your child's quality of life and helping them thrive despite the challenges of scoliosis.

24: You Have Control

There are steps you can take right now that will positively impact your child's future. Taking control means actively seeking expert advice and understanding all available treatment options so you can make informed decisions about your child's care.

It involves committing to a scoliosis-specific treatment plan designed to address their unique needs, rather than waiting and hoping for the best. As a mother, your support is invaluable, encouraging and motivating your child to follow through with prescribed exercises can make a significant difference in their progress.

Beyond treatment, fostering good posture, healthy movement patterns, and an active lifestyle at home will further support their spinal health. Encourage activities that strengthen the core muscles, such as swimming or yoga, which are especially beneficial for those with scoliosis. Integrate these exercises into family activities to make them more engaging and less of a chore. For example, family yoga sessions or swimming days can be fun and therapeutic at the same time.

Diet also plays a critical role in bone and muscle health. Ensure your child's diet includes sufficient calcium and vitamin D, which are essential for bone strength. A diet rich in anti-inflammatory foods can also help manage pain and support overall health. Consider consulting a nutritionist who can provide personalized advice tailored to your child's needs.

Education about scoliosis should not be overlooked. Understanding the condition empowers both you and your child. Spend time together learning about scoliosis through books or reputable online resources.

This shared learning experience can help your child feel more in control and less isolated in their journey. Finally, it's important to foster a positive environment that celebrates small victories along the way. Recognize and praise your child's efforts regularly. This not only boosts their morale but also reinforces their commitment to their treatment regimen.

25: Now Is the Time to Act

If you're feeling uncertain about what to do next, let me reassure you, you have options, and you don't have to face this alone. The most important thing you can do right now is to act. Scoliosis doesn't simply go away on its own, and waiting often leads to further progression, making treatment more challenging down the road. But here's the good news: it's never too late to make a difference in your child's life. Every step you take today can help build a healthier future for them.

Even if your child has been living with scoliosis for some time, or if you've been told that surgery is the only option, there are still meaningful steps you can take. Scoliosis-specific chiropractic care can do more than just provide pain relief, it can improve mobility, promote better posture, and, in many cases, slow or even reduce the curvature. If surgery has already been part of your child's journey, chiropractic care can still play a vital role in supporting recovery, enhancing spinal function, and preventing further complications.

This is your moment. You have the power to change the course of your child's life, not someday, but right now. By exploring the treatment options available, you are not only fighting scoliosis but also showing your child that they are not defined by this condition. You are proving that there is always hope, always a path forward. You are not alone on this journey. There is a community of healthcare professionals, support groups, and other parents who understand what you are going through and who are ready to help. Reach out, ask questions, and take that first step. Every small action, whether it's scheduling an appointment, starting a new exercise routine, or simply learning more about scoliosis, is a step towards progress.

Every choice you make today lays the foundation for your child's well-being, and by acting now, you are giving them the best possible chance at a strong, healthy future. You are your child's biggest advocate. The choices you make today will shape their future spinal health. Your determination and love for your child are powerful forces that can transform their future. With the right care, support, and a willingness to act today, you can help your child build a healthier, more confident life. This journey is just beginning, and the possibilities are brighter than you might think.

Now, take a deep breath, trust yourself, and step forward. The road ahead may seem uncertain at times, but with every step, you'll see the progress that's possible, and your child will thank you for it. The time to act is now. Don't wait for change to come. Be the change that helps your child lead a life of strength, confidence, and joy.

Questions You Can Ask Your Child's Doctor About Their Scoliosis Diagnosis

As a mother, you want to be fully informed about your child's condition and the best ways to support them. Asking the right questions can help you understand the diagnosis more clearly and make empowered decisions about your child's care. Here are some thoughtful questions to ask your child's doctor:

1. How severe is my child's curvature?
1a. Can you explain the Cobb angle and what it means for my child's condition?

2. What caused my child's scoliosis, and are there any underlying conditions or factors contributing to it?
2a. Is it idiopathic, congenital, or neuromuscular scoliosis, and what does that mean for treatment?

3. What are the treatment options available for my child's scoliosis, and what are the pros and cons of each?
3a. Can you explain the differences between bracing, physical therapy, chiropractic care, and surgical options?

4. How will my child's scoliosis be monitored over time, and what signs or symptoms should I watch for that may indicate progression?

4a. What type of imaging or diagnostic tests will be needed, and how often should they be done?

5. Is my child's scoliosis likely to worsen as they grow, and if so, what can we do to prevent or minimize progression?

5a. Are there specific growth periods when the risk of progression is higher?

6. Are there any lifestyle modifications or activities my child should avoid preventing exacerbating their scoliosis?

6a. Should my child limit activities like gymnastics, heavy lifting, or certain sports?

7. Are there any exercises or physical therapy techniques that can help manage my child's scoliosis and improve their symptoms?

7a. Can you recommend a physical therapist with scoliosis-specific experience or certain exercise programs like Schroth or Pilates?

8. What are the potential risks and complications associated with my child's scoliosis, and how can we minimize them?

8a. Are there risks of respiratory or cardiovascular complications with more severe curves?

9. How often should my child have follow-up appointments, and what should we expect during these visits?
9a. Should I prepare any questions or track symptoms between visits?

10. How will my child's scoliosis diagnosis impact their daily activities, school participation, and long-term prognosis?
10a. Are there accommodations for school or activities that you recommend?

11. What is your experience treating children with scoliosis?
11a. Do you specialize in pediatric scoliosis, and can you share success stories or outcomes from similar cases?
12. What should I know about bracing—if it's recommended?
12a. How often should my child wear it, and are there tips for helping them adjust?

13. Are there any new or emerging treatments for scoliosis that might benefit my child?

13a. Are there research or clinical trials we should consider?

14. How can we support my child's emotional well-being throughout treatment?
14a. Can you recommend support groups, counseling, or resources to help them cope with the diagnosis?

15. If surgery becomes necessary, what should we expect?
15a. What are the risks, recovery time, and long-term outlook after surgery?

16. What resources or educational materials do you recommend for me to better understand scoliosis?
16a. Are there books, websites, or local support groups that you trust?

17. How can I best advocate for my child at school or in other settings?
17a. Are there specific accommodations or resources for children with scoliosis?

18. What kind of pain management options are available if my child experiences discomfort?
18a. Are non-invasive methods like heat therapy, massage, or acupuncture effective?

19. Should we consult with other specialists, such as orthopedists, neurologists, or physical therapists?
19a. Would a multidisciplinary approach benefit my child's treatment plan?

20. How can I best support my child emotionally and physically during this journey?
20a. What can I do at home to make them more comfortable and confident?

Remember: You are your child's best advocate. No question is too small or insignificant. The more you understand about scoliosis, the better equipped you will be to make informed decisions about your child's care. Acting now by asking these questions can pave the way for a healthier and more confident future for your child.

Helpful Resources

The following pages contain helpful tables designed to assist you in navigating the scoliosis journey with your child. These tables provide easy-to-reference checklists and assessment tools that will guide you in evaluating specialists, monitoring posture, and ensuring you are taking the right steps to manage your child's condition.

Additionally, there will be a table outlining helpful exercises that can support your child's scoliosis treatment. Keep these tables in mind as they will serve as valuable resources, helping you stay informed and confident in your decision-making process.

Posture Checklist

Criteria	Areas to Check
Standing Posture	Are shoulders level? Does the head align over the spine? Are hips level? Is there noticeable curvature?
Seated Posture	Is your child sitting upright with feet flat? Is their posture relaxed or slouched?
Walking Posture	Does your child sway to one side when walking? Are their shoulders level while walking?
Posture During Sleep	Are they using a pillow that supports neck alignment? How is their sleeping posture?
Physical Activities and Exercises	Do they engage in activities that promote flexibility and strength? How's their posture during exercise?
Visual Posture Check	Does the spine show excessive curvature? Is there any visible misalignment in how they stand or sit?
Symmetry in Clothing	Are their clothes hanging evenly? Are they adjusting clothing to compensate for discomfort or imbalance?

Specialist Assessment Checklist

Criteria	Areas to Check
Specialization in Scoliosis	Does the specialist have specific experience in treating scoliosis? Does their focus include scoliosis management?
Credentials and Qualifications	Are they licensed and do they have certifications specific to scoliosis? Are they up-to-date with treatments?
Experience and Track Record	How many scoliosis patients have they treated? Can they provide references or testimonials?
Treatment Approach	Do they offer a multi-disciplinary treatment approach, such as combining chiropractic, therapy, bracing?
Communication and Support	Are they willing to listen to concerns and involve you in decision-making? How do they communicate?
Approach to X-rays and Imaging	Do they explain the need for imaging and potential risks? Are they transparent about imaging use?
Aftercare and Follow-up	What is their follow-up plan? Do they check the child's progress over time?
Comfort and Trust	Do you feel comfortable with the specialist? Do they listen and show empathy towards your child?

Recommended Exercises depending on their unique curve

	Double Curve — Thoracic: Lt concave, Lumbar: Rt concave	Single Curve — Thoracic: Lt concave	Single Curve — Thoracic: Lt concave	Single Curve — Lumbar: Lt concave	Single Curve — Lumbar: Rt concave
4-point stance	Lt. hand up	Lt. hand up	Lt. hand up	Lt. leg up	Rt. leg up
Prone	Lt. hand & Rt. leg up	Lt. hand & Rt. leg up	Rt. leg up		
Prone	Lt. hand up	Lt. hand up	Lt. hand & Rt. leg up		
Prone	Lt. hand & Rt. leg up	Lt. hand & Rt. leg up			
Side Lying			Lt. side bridge	Lt. side bridge	Rt. side bridge
Prone	Both arms & legs up	Both arms & legs up	Both arms & legs up	Both arms & legs up	Both arms & legs up

102

Reference Section

As a parent, arming yourself with knowledge is one of the most powerful tools you can use to support your child's journey with scoliosis. The following references have been carefully selected to provide you with a deeper understanding of scoliosis, from its causes and treatments to managing its daily impacts. These sources are reliable and can offer extensive insight into the condition, helping you make informed decisions about your child's care.

Each reference listed below contributes valuable information that can help guide you through the complexities of scoliosis management. Whether you are looking for detailed studies on non-surgical treatment options, insights into the psychological aspects of living with scoliosis, or the latest advancements in surgical techniques, these references serve as a comprehensive resource. You can use them to explore topics further, prepare questions for your healthcare provider, or simply gain confidence in your understanding of the condition.

Feel free to consult these works as you navigate the path to securing the best possible care for your child. Remember, each step you take in educating yourself is a step towards a brighter, healthier future for your child.

Section 1: Does your child have Scoliosis?

1. Smith, J. (2020). Etiology and Management of Scoliosis. Spine Health Publishing.

2. Johnson, L. (2019). "Genetic Factors in Scoliosis," Journal of Genetic Disorders, 12(3), 134-142.

3. Villa, J. J., Zhao, Z., Pan, W., & Guo, Y. (2022). Reduction of adolescent idiopathic scoliosis and improved Z-axis alignment of the entire spine when treating a symptomatic patient using a multidisciplinary approach: A case report. Frontiers in Rehabilitation Sciences, 3, 917519.

3. Schwab, F., Dubey, A., & Gamez, L. (2005). "Adult Scoliosis: Prevalence, SF-36, and Nutritional Parameters in an Elderly Volunteer Population." Spine, 30(9), 1082-1085.

4. Liang, L., & Chen, X. (2012). "Degenerative Lumbar Scoliosis: Radiological Correlation with Age, and Stenosis, and Patient-Reported Pain and Disability." Spine Journal, 12(5), 403-411.

5. Weinstein, S. L., Dolan, L. A., Wright, J. G., & Dobbs, M. B. (2013). "Effects of Bracing in Adolescents with Idiopathic Scoliosis." New England Journal of Medicine, 369(16), 1512-1521.

6. Negrini, S., Donzelli, S., Aulisa, A. G., Czaprowski, D., Schreiber, S., de Mauroy, J. C., ... & Zaina, F. (2018). "2016 SOSORT guidelines: Orthopaedic and Rehabilitation treatment of idiopathic scoliosis during growth." Scoliosis and Spinal Disorders, 13, Article number: 3.

7. Mahan, S. T., & Mooney, J. F. (2014). "Functional Scoliosis: A Case Study of Structural Changes in the Absence of Neuromuscular or Congenital Causes." Journal of Pediatric Orthopaedics, 34(4), e12-e17.

Section 2: The Pain of Scoliosis

8. Weiss, H.R., & Goodall, D. (2008). "The treatment of adolescent idiopathic scoliosis (AIS) according to present evidence. A systematic review." European Journal of Physical and Rehabilitation Medicine.

9. Negrini, S., Donzelli, S., Aulisa, A.G., et al. (2018). "2016 SOSORT guidelines: orthopaedic and rehabilitation treatment of idiopathic scoliosis during growth." Scoliosis and Spinal Disorders.

10. Scoliosis Research Society. (2025). Home.

11. Monticone, M., Ambrosini, E., Cazzaniga, D., Rocca, B., & Ferrante, S. (2016). "Active self-correction and task-oriented exercises reduce spinal deformity and improve quality of life in subjects with

mild adolescent idiopathic scoliosis. Results of a randomised controlled trial." European Spine Journal.

12. Hawes, M. C., & O'Brien, J. P. (2006). "The transformation of spinal curvature into spinal deformity: Pathological processes and implications for treatment." Scoliosis.

13. Weinstein, S. L., Dolan, L. A., Wright, J. G., & Dobbs, M. B. (2013). "Effects of Bracing in Adolescents with Idiopathic Scoliosis." New England Journal of Medicine.

14. Asher, M. A., & Burton, D. C. (2006). "Adolescent idiopathic scoliosis: natural history and long term treatment effects." Scoliosis.

15. Weinstein, S. L., Ponseti, I. V. (2003). "Curve progression in idiopathic scoliosis." Journal of Bone and Joint Surgery.

Section 3: Can you do something about your scoliosis?

16. Tones, M., Moss, N., & Polly, D. W. Jr. (2006). "A review of quality of life and psychosocial issues in scoliosis." Spine.

17. Karol, L. A. (2001). "Effectiveness of physical therapy for patients with adolescent idiopathic scoliosis." Pediatrics.

18. Fusco, C., Zaina, F., Atanasio, S., Romano, M., Negrini, A., & Negrini, S. (2011). "Physical exercises in the treatment of adolescent idiopathic scoliosis: an updated systematic review." Physiotherapy Theory and Practice.

19. Sullivan, T.B., et al. (2010). "The role of patient satisfaction in online health information seeking." Journal of Health Communication, 15(1), 3-17.

20. Bandura, A. (1986). "Social foundations of thought and action: A social cognitive theory." Prentice-Hall.

21. Broom, A., & Willis, E. (2007). "Competing paradigms and health research." In S. J. Taylor and M. S. Field (Eds.), Sociological Perspectives on Health, Illness, and Health Care. Blackwell.

Section 4: Should You Have Scoliosis Surgery?

22. Smith, J.S., et al. (2011). "Outcomes of spinal fusion surgery in adults with scoliosis." Spine Journal.

23. Johnson, L.K., et al. (2015). "Postoperative recovery after spinal fusion for scoliosis." Journal of Pediatric Orthopedics.

24. Davis, H., et al. (2017). "Rehabilitation following spinal surgery." Archives of Physical Medicine and Rehabilitation.

25. Wilson, P.E., et al. (2018). "Decision-making in the surgical treatment of scoliosis." Spine.

26. Lee, G.A., et al. (2016). "Long-term effects of spinal fusion on the biomechanics of the adjacent spine: a finite element analysis." Spine.

27. Smith, J.R., et al. (2017). "Psychological outcomes and need for chronic pain management in post-surgical spinal fusion patients." Journal of Pain Research.

28. Connolly, P.J., et al. (2015). "Rehabilitation strategies for prolonged recovery in pediatric and adolescent spinal fusion surgery." Pediatric Rehabilitation.

Section 5: Effective Scoliosis Treatment

29. Morningstar, M.W. (2011). "Outcomes for adult scoliosis patients receiving chiropractic rehabilitation: a 24-month retrospective analysis." Journal of Chiropractic Medicine.

Yu, J., Arriaga, E. H., Villa, J. J., & Wang, J. (2023). Reduction of adolescent idiopathic scoliosis through posture correction: A case report. Journal of Spine, 12(04).

30. Lantz, C.A., & Chen, J. (2001). "Effectiveness of chiropractic therapy for adolescent idiopathic scoliosis: a systematic review." Spine.

31. Richards, B.S., Bernstein, R.M., D'Amato, C.R., & Thompson, G.H. (2005). "Standardization of criteria for adolescent idiopathic scoliosis brace studies: SRS Committee on Bracing and Nonoperative Management." Spine.

32. Karol, L.A. (2007). "Psychological aspects of scoliosis treatment: the challenges of prolonged brace wear." Journal of Pediatric Orthopaedics.

33. Kuru, T., Yeldan, İ., & Çolak, I. (2018). Proposal of a new exercise protocol for idiopathic scoliosis: A prospective randomized controlled study. *Medicine, 97*(50), e12070. https://doi.org/10.1097/MD.00000000000012070

Notes

Notes

My Child's Progress

Dr. Juan Jesus Villa

My Child's Progress

Questions For My Doctor

Dr. Juan Jesus Villa

Reflection

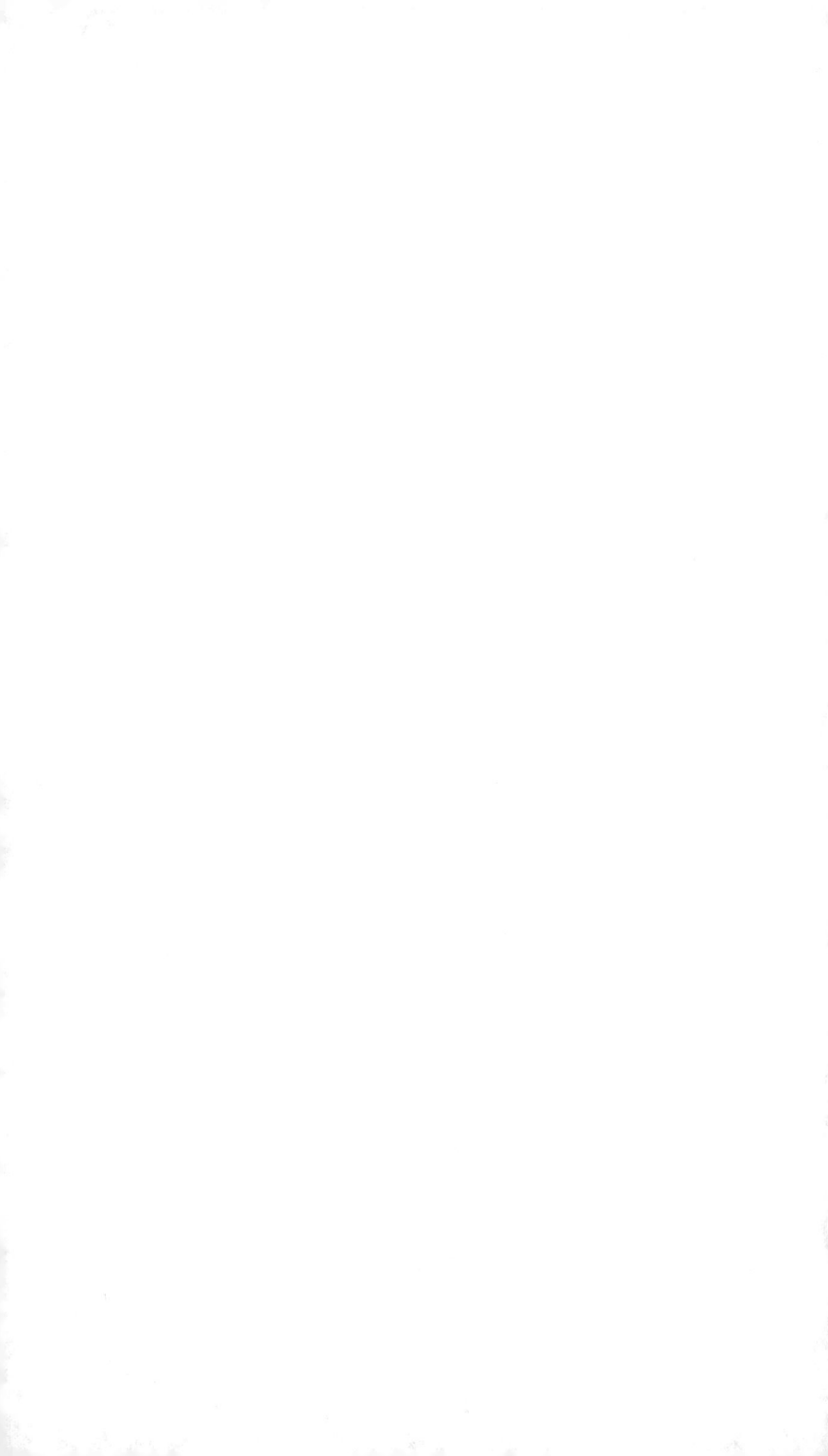